ABOUT THE AU

Maryon Stewart studied preventive
St George's Hospital in London a
with nutritional doctors in England for four years. At the
beginning of 1984 she set up the PMT Advisory Service which
has subsequently helped thousands of women world-wide. In
1987 she launched the Women's Nutritional Advisory Service,
which now provides broader help to women of all ages.

Maryon Stewart is the author of the best-selling books *The
Zest for Life Plan*, *The Phyto Factor*, *Cruising through the Menopause*,
No More PMS, now in its third edition, *Beat Sugar Craving* and
Healthy Parents, Healthy Baby. She is the co-author of *No More
IBS*, *Beat PMS Cookbook* and *Every Woman's Health Guide*. Her
new book *The Natural Health Bible* was published this year.

She has worked extensively on radio including a weekly
radio programme of her own on health and nutrition, has co-
written several medical papers and has written for many glossy
magazines and for the national daily newspapers. She has also
appeared on many TV programmes on all five channels, radio
programmes and had a regular page in *House & Garden* and
Healthy Eating as well as a column in the *Sunday Express
Magazine*. She has been both advisor and contributor to *Good
Health Magazine*, on the Expert Panel for *Top Sante* magazine
and writes regularly for ThinkNatural.com and Beme.com.
She is currently the nutritional consultant for a new Channel
4 programme entitled *Model Behaviour*. She was voted one of
the most influential women of Great Britain by *Good
Housekeeping* magazine. She frequently lectures to both the
public and medical profession. She is married to Dr Alan
Stewart; they live in Lewes, Sussex, with their four children.

... dentistry and nutrition at ... until recently, and worked as a counsellor

The Model Plan

Eating well
Looking good
Feeling great

Maryon Stewart

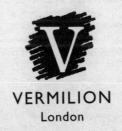

VERMILION
London

1 3 5 7 9 10 8 6 4 2

Text copyright © Maryon Stewart 2001

First published in the United Kingdom in 2001 by Vermilion
an imprint of Ebury Press
Random Rouse, 20 Vauxhall Bridge Road, London SW1V 2SA

Random House Australia (Pty) Limited
20 Alfred Street, Milsons Point, Sydney, New South Wales 2061, Australia

Random House New Zealand Limited
18 Poland Road, Glenfield, Auckland 10, New Zealand

Random House South Africa (Pty) Limited
Endulini, 5A Jubilee Road, Parktown 2193, South Africa

Random House UK Limited Reg. No.954009

A CIP catalogue record for this book is available from the British Library

ISBN: 0 09 188242 7

Printed and bound in Great Britain by Bookmarque Ltd, Croydon, Surrey.

Papers used by Vermilion are natural, recyclable products made from wood
grown in sustainable forests.

'Enough is as good as a feast'

To Rosa Kingston and Mary Stewart, my mother and mother-in-law, with love and appreciation – you never dreamed that your lessons would have such far reaching implications!

Acknowledgements

Although I am technically the author of this book, as always, putting it together has truly been a team effort, and it's time for the team to take a bow.

My first thanks must go to Dr Alan Stewart, my husband, not only for his contribution to the book itself, but for being so supportive generally, and making it possible for me to 'go missing' at home in order to get the book written out of hours.

My next pat on the back goes to Helen Heap, our nutritionist, for her help with the diet section and the appendix. It would have been a whole lot harder without her help.

As ever, I am forever indebted to my patients over the last 18 years, who have given me the clinical experience needed to write with authority. I want to also say a particular thank you to those who agreed to share their stories with you in this book – I have changed their names, but not at their request for they are all willing to talk freely about their experiences.

My next vote of thanks goes to Cheryl Griffiths, our office manageress, for keeping the show on the road while I was preoccupied, and to the team at the WNAS, in particular Lisa Graham, Janet Pratt, Terri Hennessy and Shirley Campbell, for their ongoing support.

I am also incredibly grateful to Madeleine Knight and her team at Princess Productions for inviting me to work on *Model Behaviour*; it has been a unique experience!

My gratitude also goes to Amelia Thorpe and Kate Adams at Vermilion for their foresight and encouragement, and to Charlotte Howard, my Literary Agent, for being such a professional.

Credit and heartfelt thanks must go also to Dr Lucia

Capachione, for sharing her experiences and wisdom, so enabling me to focus on designing life my way.

On the home front, thanks go to Gill Boyall, for keeping the house running efficiently, and to Claire Baker and Liz Copping for entertaining our two youngest children in my absence.

I would sincerely like to thank the children themselves, Phoebe, Chesney, Hester and Simeon for so willingly giving me the space to get on with the book, and putting their own needs on hold.

And, finally, whoever arranged for the sun to shine while I wrote, and the inventor of the laptop, should not go unacknowledged. Being able to soak up some sunshine while I worked has been an added bonus.

Contents

INTRODUCTION

How to look good and feel better than you can remember

When I was asked to act as the nutritional consultant for the television programme *Model Behaviour* I accepted the challenge with enthusiasm. Having given advice to large numbers of young women during the 18 years I have been running the Women's Nutritional Advisory Service (WNAS), and frequently lecturing to groups of students, I felt incredibly well qualified. I knew that I would be looking after the nutritional welfare of a group of young women, and that they would probably have only basic skills in that department.

In reality, their lack of knowledge about the needs of their body, how to put together a simple shopping list based on a menu plan, or prepare even basic food, was a bit of an eye-opener. It brought home to me the devastating effects of the lack of knowledge about the basics of how to feed and care for yourself, because I am only too aware of the consequences. My own children have all learned to shop for and prepare basic food because these activities have been an inbuilt part of their lives. My work with the girls on *Model Behaviour* made me realise that, as health and nutrition are no longer compulsory subjects in the National Curriculum, unless the lessons had been learned at home these skills were altogether a missing part of their education.

Instead, being more concerned with looking like Giselle or Kate Moss has become far more fashionable than meeting the nutritional needs of the body. Many young people have become obsessed with looking good, and will often starve themselves to get into the shape they have been persuaded by the advertising industry to be ideal, or alternatively skip proper meals and snack on junk food instead. However, unbeknown to them, due to lack of education, they do so at the expense of both their physical and mental health as well as their appearance.

The desire to look good coupled with the temptation to live on both junk and fast food, and a lack of knowledge about meeting the needs of the body, have lead to disastrous consequences. A recent government survey of 15 to 18 year olds, published in 2000, produced some pretty damning evidence to show that nutritional trouble is on the horizon. When their diets were analysed a high percentage were found to have intakes that were below the minimum recommended amounts for several minerals. For example, intake of iron was low in 54 per cent of cases, magnesium in 53 per cent, and calcium and zinc in 19 per cent and 10 per cent of cases respectively. From blood tests it was estimated that up to 95 per cent of the sample had low vitamin B2 levels, 15 per cent low zinc levels, 8 per cent had low vitamin A intake and 26 per cent of girls had low iron stores.

The nutritional deficiencies outlined affect most aspects of health and result in all sorts of symptoms including premenstrual syndrome, mood swings, headaches, acne, irritable bowel syndrome, fatigue, period problems, cravings for food, lack of concentration and depression. In addition, the condition of hair, skin and nails in general will be detrimentally affected.

I didn't have to be a rocket scientist to realise that there was a desperate need for a simple self-help book, so that those who have missed out can get genned up on the basics of not only how to look good, but also how to continue to be healthy in both the short- and long-term, in an enjoyable and practical way.

Diet is an important part of the missing education, but it doesn't end there. Lifestyle, including exercise, relaxation, social substances and even self-esteem and faith in your abilities to achieve well in life, are all topics on the list of what's missing from our education. The cogs of my mind went into overdrive, and the concept for *The Model Plan* was born.

The Model Plan is your very own workbook, which contains details of how to keep your body in good shape on the inside as well as enhancing the bits that show. I have written it in bite-sized sections, with plenty of practical self-help, plus hints, tips, and case histories. There are also questionnaires to complete in order to assess your needs. Part One will provide you with education about meeting your body's needs. You will learn how to interpret the messages sent by your body and by the end of the book it is highly likely that you will know much more about the effects of diet on your health and your physical appearance than your own doctor.

In Part Two I have covered many of the common problems we experience, including skin problems, gut troubles, troublesome periods, headaches, thrush and fatigue, each with a detailed self-help section based on 18 years of clinical experience and a wealth of published medical research. This section will arm you with the tools to help you to focus on choosing the right direction in your life, rather than waiting for things to happen or just accepting what comes your way, as well as boosting your self-esteem beyond belief.

In addition to the Healthy Eating Plan, which you will find in Part Three, there is also a big section on the Discovery Diet, which will enable you to conduct an experiment on your body to find the right kind of diet for your particular needs. There are suggested simple menu plans and even some simple but delicious recipes for you to try out. You will also have the opportunity to record and write your own programme from the information you collect as you go through the book.

In Part Four you will find your daily diaries, information on the nutritional content of particular foods, and a directory entitled Good Food – Where to Find It and lists of Healthy Shopping Options. So it couldn't be simpler. All you need to do is browse through the sections that you feel will be of most interest, completing the questionnaires and working out your scores as you go along.

I have enjoyed my work with the girls on *Model Behaviour* immensely, and you too can now benefit from my experience, for I had the opportunity to try out the set of recommendations that are now contained in *The Model Plan*, and fine-tune them as I went along.

You are about to go on a most enjoyable voyage of discovery that will pay great dividends both now and in the longer term. As a result of your new knowledge you will look better, feel healthier and get far more out of what may even turn out to be a longer life.

Enjoy!

Maryon Stewart
October 2001

PART ONE

Look Fab, Feel Great

CHAPTER I

Beware the effects of diet on health and beauty

Looking good and feeling well is not a gift to us from Mother Nature, but an acquired skill. The minority of us who are born with a perfect figure, gorgeous hair and clear skin may have to put in less effort, but in reality we all have to work at preserving our health and beauty. Sadly, we are born with a design fault, which means that our body has specific needs in order to continue to serve us well and to look good. Most of us know that too many parties with alcohol on tap, skipped meals and too little sleep will eventually start to tell visual tales, for our diet and lifestyle affect every essence of our being, including how we look as well as how we feel.

Food is probably the last thing on your mind at a time when you are concentrating on looking good. However, to be able to present yourself well and meet the demands that will undoubtedly be placed upon you in life, you will need to learn how to look after your body properly.

The inadequacy of our diet

Amazingly the human body is terrific at communicating what it likes and dislikes, and also lets us know when our nutritional needs are not being met. Sadly few of us learn about the importance of good nutrition at any stage of our education, which is probably why so many of us are suffering from poor dietary habits and even nutritional deficiencies that affect us both physically and mentally.

Recent government surveys show clearly that young people are often short of nutrients like iron, zinc, calcium, magnesium and certain B vitamins. These deficiencies not only affect the way we feel, they also affect the way we look. Common problems like acne spots, greasy skin, cracking at the corners of the mouth, red patches at the side of the nose, pimples on the upper arms or thighs, unmanageable hair and split brittle nails all have a nutritional story to tell.

Beauty from within

I have prepared a chart which outlines some of the deficiencies so that you can better understand the needs of your body. Have a close look – you will be amazed by how many signs there are.

Realizing that you may be short of certain nutrients is the first step. The next step is putting it right. And it's not just a question of taking a pill, for it's important to know which foods and drinks will provide the nutrients you require and, likewise, which foods and drinks may interfere with the absorption of good nutrients.

Keeping the demons at bay

As well as the obvious physical signs, the body needs plenty of good nutrients in order to serve you well. If you have ever felt tired for no apparent reason or have experienced period problems or premenstrual syndrome, or had a sudden outbreak of spots, or episodes of digestive problems, you will understand that your well-being may not always have been under your control. However, it's extremely likely that the underlying problem is related to your diet.

During the course of *The Model Plan* I will be teaching you about healthy eating and how to detect and correct nutritional

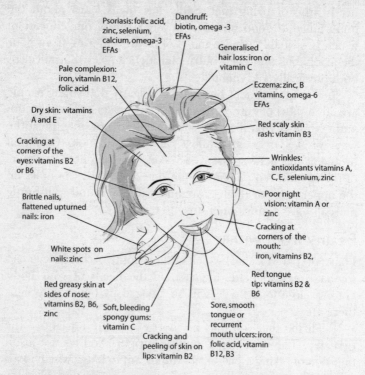

Psoriasis: folic acid, zinc, selenium, calcium, omega-3 EFAs

Dandruff: biotin, omega -3 EFAs

Generalised hair loss: iron or vitamin C

Pale complexion: iron, vitamin B12, folic acid

Eczema: zinc, B vitamins, omega-6 EFAs

Dry skin: vitamins A and E

Red scaly skin rash: vitamin B3

Cracking at corners of the eyes: vitamins B2 or B6

Wrinkles: antioxidants vitamins A, C, E, selenium, zinc

Brittle nails, flattened upturned nails: iron

Poor night vision: vitamin A or zinc

Cracking at corners of the mouth: iron, vitamins B2,

White spots on nails: zinc

Red tongue tip: vitamins B2 & B6

Red greasy skin at sides of nose: vitamins B2, B6, zinc

Soft, bleeding spongy gums: vitamin C

Sore, smooth tongue or recurrent mouth ulcers: iron, folic acid, vitamin B12, B3

Cracking and peeling of skin on lips: vitamin B2

Some physical features of vitamin & mineral deficiencies

deficiencies, so that you have the tools at your fingertips to keep feeling well, with plenty of energy and with your good looks positively glowing.

Nutritious vs. not so nutritious

Most of you probably know that it is better to eat a wholesome meal than a chocolate bar or a sticky bun. But the clever advertising industry works hard to convince us that fast food, chocolate and cola-based drinks, for example, will make us feel good as well as making us attractive to others. Rather than falling for the hype, it is important for you to be able to look at the facts and recognize a myth when it presents itself.

Let's take the example of two different meals. The first is a pasta dish with tomato sauce and parmesan cheese, followed by fruit sorbet. The second is fresh salmon with potatoes, broccoli and carrots, followed by bananas with nuts and ice-cream. The drinks with the pasta meal are cola and coffee, and the drinks with the fish meal are fruit juice and herb tea.

You could be forgiven for thinking that these two meals are equally nutritious. However, the fish meal is the winner in terms of nutritional content. This is a good example, because pasta has become very popular and is perceived to be nutritious, when in fact it is a processed carbohydrate. The fish meal offers much more protein, essential fatty acids and vitamins and minerals, all of which are important to both your health and your appearance.

The desserts also are poles apart in terms of nutritional content. The ice-cream, banana and nuts will provide the body with lots more goodies, especially calcium and vitamin B, than the sorbet, which is mainly composed of a little fruit juice, sugar and water. As for the drinks, the fruit juice provides vitamin C as well as other good nutrients, while the cola contains lots of sugar, caffeine and chemicals that limit the absorption of calcium. Fruit tea is preferable to coffee, as coffee contains caffeine which can over-stimulate our systems, and in excess can leave us feeling nervous, panicky and unable to sleep.

These days many of us are lacking culinary or kitchen skills, as we no longer learn to cook at school, so unless one of our parents is a keen cook, the chances are we are out there with the rest of them looking for fast, easy options.

Get into shape without dieting

All this is talk of food, when many of you may be thinking of shedding a few pounds to enhance your appearance. Well, the good news is that you can consume a healthy diet without gaining weight, and regular exercise will help to increase the rate at which your metabolism ticks over, so that you burn up the calories.

Believe it or not 50 years ago we were eating three or four proper meals each day with one between-meal snack, whereas today, we have on average one proper meal per day with three or four snacks. You may justifiably ask why the nation wasn't fatter 50 years ago. The answer is probably that we did far more exercise, mostly relying on our legs to get us around rather than cars or buses. Many of us are now dealing with the consequences these dietary and lifestyle changes have inflicted upon our general health as well as on the shape and size of our bodies.

The key to maintaining your weight is to learn to meet your body's needs, which includes finding the right kind of diet for your individual body and keeping your metabolic rate ticking over with regular exercise. Very often it is not how much we consume but the kind of food we eat that determines our weight and how we feel.

During the course of the book you will be able to explore the areas of diet and lifestyle so that you can find the right plan to keep you looking good, while at the same time helping to maximise your energy and keep you feeling in the peak of health. The Discovery Diet which you will find on page 172, is an eight-week plan based on 18 years of research at the WNAS. In addition, you will have the opportunity to overcome common troubles like premenstrual syndrome, problems with your periods or your skin, digestive upsets or simply cravings for sweet food should you have them. You will be able to plan out what you should be aiming to eat for each meal, and for those of you who can't cook, you will find a series of really simple menus that don't involve much preparation. I will give you all the secret nutritious short cuts that I have discovered over the last 18 years so that you can keep it simple, but still reap the benefits of a nutritious diet and wholesome lifestyle.

CHAPTER 2

Is your diet good for you?

Most people are fortunate enough to be able to eat when they are hungry, without giving too much thought to what they are actually eating. As long as it fills the gap and relieves the pangs of hunger, that's fine. Some even eat when they are not hungry, perhaps as a comfort, through boredom or because they particularly like the taste of a certain kind of food – like chocolate, for example.

I want you to read through the questionnaire that follows and tick the boxes that most apply to your eating habits.

This may be the first time you have been asked to stop and analyse your diet. Be absolutely honest, as you won't be fooling anyone except yourself. Once you have finished marking the questionnaire work out your score and read through the results. If you did really well you can pat both yourself and your parents on the back, because it is likely that the example you were set at home has rubbed off on you. If on the other hand you don't do so well, take comfort in the fact that you are about to gain some amazing knowledge as you go through *The Model Plan*, which will more than make up for anything you haven't learned before.

Is your diet good for you?

Tick the circle most relevant to your consumption in each category.

Cows milk: full cream or semi-skimmed
a 2 litres or more per week ○
b 1–2 litres per week ○
c Less than 1 litre per week ○

Soya milk – calcium fortified
a 2 litres or more per week ○
b 1–2 litres per week ○
c Less than 1 litre per week ○

Cheese
a 125–250g per week ○
b 50–124g per week ○
c 0–49g per week ○

Eggs
a 3–6 per week ○
b 1–2 per week ○
c None ○

Main meal with protein (animal or vegetarian)
a Every day ○
b 5 or 6 per week ○
c 4 or fewer per week ○

Breakfast
a Every day ○
b 5 or 6 per week ○
c 4 or fewer per week ○

Fruit, vegetables and salad
a 5 or more servings per day ○
b 3–4 servings per day ○
c 2 servings or fewer per day ○

Tea and coffee
a 0–2 mugs per day ○
b 3–5 mugs per day ○
c 6 mugs or more per day ○

Alcohol
a 1 drink per day (fewer than 10 units per week) ○
b 8–14 drinks per week (11–20 units) ○
c 15 drinks per week (21 units or more) ○

Cola based drinks: non-diet and diet
a 0–1 per week ○
b 2–3 per week ○
c 4 or more ○

Chocolate bars or equivalent
a 0–1 bars per week ○
b 2–3 bars per week ○
c 4 or more per week ○

Biscuits
a 0–4 per week ○
b 5–14 per week ○
c 15 or more ○

Cakes and puddings
a 0–2 per week ○
b 3–5 per week ○
c 6 or more ○

Sweets

a 0–1 per day ○
b 2–3 per day ○
c 4 or more ○

Teaspoons of sugar added to tea or coffee

a None ○
b ½–1 teaspoon ○
c 1 or more ○

Pizza & Pasta

a 0–1 servings per week ○
b 2–3 servings per week ○
c 4 or more servings per week ○

Packets of crisps

a 0 –1 per week ○
b 2 – 3 per week ○
c 4 or more per week ○

Salt added in cooking or at the table

a Never ○
b Occasionally ○
c Regularly ○

Fish

a 2 or more servings per week ○
b 1 serving per week ○
c Never ○

Lean red meat

a 3–5 portions per week ○
b Less than 2 or more than 5 portions per week ○
c 1 or none ○

Sausage, pies and bacon

a 0–3 times per week ○
b 4–5 times per week ○
c 6 or more times per week ○

Take-aways (burger, Chinese, Indian, fried chicken, fish & chips)

a 0–1 per week ○
b 2 per week ○
c 3 or more per week ○

Fresh potatoes (not chips)

a 4 or more times per week ○
b 2–3 times per week ○
c 1 or fewer per week ○

Skip a meal

a Never ○
b 1–2 per week ○
c 3 or more ○

a Optimum . . . .
b Dodgy . . . .
c Really Bad . . . .

Your score

- If you scored 18 or more ticks against the As you are doing really well with your diet.
- A score of 13–17 As means that you are not doing too badly, but there is room for improvement.
- If you have a score of 12 or less As and everything else is B, you will need to follow the Healthy Eating Plan on page 158 and make a real effort to improve your eating habits.
- If most of your scores were Bs and Cs your diet needs a complete overhaul! You will need to read Chapter Three –

What's wrong with our diet? very carefully, taking the messages on board. Look on the positive side, because your diet has been so bad, you are likely to experience a great sense of well-being once you are through the withdrawal symptoms and consuming much healthier options.

CHAPTER 3

What's wrong with our diet?

Our food is expected to fulfil an incredible number of needs. It has to provide us with energy and essential nutrients in order to stay alive, as well as be pleasurable and serve a social function. We want it to be fast, available, tasty, convenient, predictable, sometimes even unpredictable and new, and to hell with the nutritional content! But we also want to be able to share it with friends and family, to indulge in it and use it to indulge others and for it to be a delight to our senses; a feast for our eyes, an aroma, a taste, to have good mouth appeal and even to have a satisfying sound as we crunch.

Why is it that when food can be so satisfying we are often willing to put up with second best?

Many people go for sheer quantity and convenience, regardless of the quality, which is perhaps why obesity has become a runaway problem in many developed countries. By and large we have followed the lead of the United States where, 'If one is good then two must be better'.

How much do we consume?

The answer to this simple question is in some ways easy but in other ways quite complicated. If you eat too little you lose weight and if you eat too much you gain weight. If you are underweight on a long-term basis then it is safe to assume that you've actually been eating an inadequate amount for some time, usually months or years, and vice-versa for the overweight. As more and more people at all ages are overweight then we must all be eating more and more food. Wrong! The truth is quite the opposite. Studies groups show a consistent trend over the last 50 years of declining food energy intake.

This leads us to draw the correct and inevitable conclusion that we actually need less energy from food than our parents and grandparents because we are less physically active than they were. But our needs for many vitamins and minerals are very similar regardless of energy intake. Thus in these modern times we need to obtain much the same amounts of vitamins and minerals but from a smaller amount of food. This is not easy if we also consume energy-rich foods that are very low or even devoid of any vitamins and minerals. These include most alcoholic drinks, sugar and sweet foods, fizzy drinks and many fat-rich foods.

The components of our diet

Let us now look at the different components of our diet, beginning with protein, which is the foundation to life.

Protein
Why we need it
Proteins are made up of individual amino acids which are needed for the growth and repair of tissues. Some of the essential amino acids are only found in certain foods and a relative lack of them can have profound effects upon our health. Proteins are needed by our bodies to produce many hormones, enzymes, brain chemicals, the walls of cells, hair, nails and the supporting structure for many tissues. Proteins are eventually broken down into the waste chemical urea which is passed out in the urine.

Protein comes in two main forms, animal protein which provides a very good balance of essential amino acids and vegetarian proteins which do not provide a full complement of amino acids unless two or more different protein-rich foods, such as beans and wheat, are combined.

Sugar, fats and alcohol provide no proteins and fruit and vegetables contain only small amounts. Good sources of protein are meats, liver, eggs, milk, cheese, fish and shellfish, beans, nuts and seeds, soya and tofu. It is important that the main meal each day contains an adequate portion of protein and that the other meals also provide a modest amount. Increased amounts of protein are needed in those who are more physically active, are pregnant or breastfeeding, are growing, or needing to put on weight after an illness.

Protein should provide between 10 and 15 per cent of the calories we consume and having a long-term intake below this can be unhealthy.

Protein deficiency

Most people in the UK do quite well for protein. Too much protein is almost never a problem but in the United States high protein levels have been linked to osteoporosis.

Too little protein can cause some substantial problems which may be long-lasting. These include:

- poor growth and development in children and teenagers
- very thin and weak muscles most noticeable on the upper arms
- poor resistance to infection
- period problems including absent periods and premenstrual syndrome with breast tenderness
- fatigue
- delayed recovery from accidents, illnesses or major operations
- associated lack of iron, zinc and vitamin B.

What you can do about it

There is plenty you can do and it doesn't take much effort. Ideally you need to have a main meal with an adequate amount of animal protein (at least 120–175 gm) each day.

During the rest of the day also have at least one of the following:
- 300ml milk *or*
- 75–100g cheese per day *or*
- 2 eggs *or*
- 75g mixed nuts or seeds.

If you are vegetarian you should have:
- at least 500ml milk or soya milk
- a main meal with either 2 eggs, 75–100g cheese or 125–150g beans, *or* 100g tofu or Quorn
- 2–4 slices wholegrain bread
- also eat one or more portions of sweetcorn, fresh or frozen peas, nuts and seeds.

Fat

Why we need 'good' fat

Yes there is 'good' fat. Yes, fat contains lots of calories and many of us eat a bit too much, but there is actually good fat, for two reasons:

1 Some fats provide essential fatty acids, of which there are two families: Omega 6 series which come from quality vegetable oils and Omega 3 series which come from vegetable and fish oils.
2 Fatty foods provide essential minerals and vitamins, especially calcium and vitamin A. These are found mainly in quality dairy foods and eggs. Eggs are good for you too, and a reasonable consumption for most people is three or four per week. Eggs are a rich source of protein, vitamin A and B and iron and they are relatively inexpensive. Free-range eggs are also a good source of the Omega 3 oils, which is tremendously important.

How much good fat do we need?

Firstly we don't need much but we do need some. These specialised fats can be burnt as fuel but can also be used to form the walls of all the cells in the body. The structure of the cell wall influences the efficiency of chemical reactions inside the cell. This is particularly true of the brain, which has a high fat content and needs these specialised essential fatty acids in order to function efficiently. Essential fatty acids have been shown to influence the rate of development of the brain in new-born babies and may also influence our behaviour, mood and the progress of some neurological disorders. Additionally these fats play a part in skin quality, helping to prevent it from drying excessively. One of the fats from the Omega 6 series, called Gamma Linolenic Acid (GLA), which is found in evening primrose oil, can be helpful for eczema, as well as for women with premenstrual breast tenderness.

The Omega 3 series contain two fats Eicosapentaenoic Acid (EPA) and Docosahexaenoic Acid (DHA), which are found in high concentrations in cod liver oil and other fish oils. They can help to reduce the severity of inflammation in those with arthritis and the chronic skin condition psoriasis.

On average adult men consume 14g of Omega 6 and 2g of Omega 3 oils, and women 10g of Omega 6 and 1.5g of Omega 3 oils, per week. By and large these figures are considered to be adequate, provided the rest of the diet is well balanced and provides the necessary vitamins and minerals, and as long as the individual does not drink alcohol excessively or smoke heavily.

Quality carbohydrate
Why we need quality carbohydrate
In the UK about 50 per cent of all our energy comes from the carbohydrates in our diet. The main food sources are bread, wheat and other grain products, sugar, fruit and vegetables and alcohol. In their natural state wholewheat and brown rice are rich not only in carbohydrate but also in many vitamins and minerals, including vitamin B and magnesium, which are needed by our bodies for the chemical reactions that allow the release of energy from the carbohydrate itself.

Now for the really important bit! In the developed world we have invented machinery that enables us to process staple foods such as wheat, rice and sugar but in doing so we lose some of these essential vitamins and minerals.

For example:
- White rice is less nutritious than brown rice which retains the tough outer coating, a rich source of vitamin B1 – thiamin.
- White flour has a much lower content of vitamin B, magnesium and iron than wholemeal flour (though white flour is fortified with vitamin B, calcium and iron).
- Sugar cane has a reasonable mineral content compared with refined white sugar, which contains no vitamins and minerals whatsoever, while brown sugar retains some of the minerals present in sugar before the refining process.

So now we have foods that are high in calories and low in essential nutrients. This isn't a problem if we eat very little of them, but in truth we eat plenty. What makes things worse is that we now eat less and less food, and cannot afford to dedicate so much of our intake to these high calorie 'empty' foods.

How much do we consume?
- On the whole men and women of all ages eat too many cakes, biscuits, puddings, sweets and chocolate. These are high in carbohydrate with some not too healthy animal fats, and low in most vitamins and minerals.
- We all like carbohydrate and most of us have a sweet tooth. Many of us like 'quick carbohydrate' which means it comes in a packet, often with refined contents, which may have a poor nutrient content.

How to improve carbohydrate intake
- First of all don't eat too much of it. Leave room for the vegetables and fruit in your diet which will provide you with lots of vitamins and minerals. You can have more

carbohydrate if you are not overweight and are exercising regularly.

- Make half your bread intake wholemeal or granary and half white. White bread isn't bad for you but try to strike a balance, unless you are following the Discovery Diet on page 172, in which case you will be cutting wheat out of your diet altogether for a while.
- Try brown rice; it needs longer to cook and it has a nutty flavour.
- Limit pasta and pizza to a maximum of one serving of each per week and preferably half this amount. You cannot beat potatoes and fresh green vegetables for carbohydrates with class.
- Watch the naughty carbohydrates – the cakes, biscuits, buns and puddings. In general the consumption of these, and of sweets and chocolate, need to be halved. Have some sugar but keep it to a minimum. Unless you are trying to lose weight, restrict eating these foods to about three to four times per week in total.

Dairy products
Why we need quality dairy products
Milk, cheese, yoghurt, cream and butter are traditional and important foods in our diets and have been a central part of good nutrition, particularly for children, for the last century. Dairy products, in particular, milk and cheese, are rich sources of:

- Protein for growth and development
- Vitamin A – retinol for growth, resistance to infection and vision
- Vitamin B2 – riboflavin for energy and to prevent lips peeling and cracking
- Calcium for healthy strong bones and teeth at all ages
- Iodine for energy and for normal function of the thyroid gland.

Dairy products came in for a knock with the 'anti-fat – lower your cholesterol' message during the eighties and nineties and so many of the traditional dairy products have fallen in consumption. We have chosen lower fat versions of milk, yoghurt and cheese, and the anti-fat lobby, together with the fizzy drinks lobby, have pushed out the dairy foods from their traditional position. Milk is no longer a daily drink at school. You are more likely to find a packet of crisps in a school lunch box than a piece of cheese or a milk-based drink, and when did you last see anyone over the age of 18 holding a glass of milk? As a result the intake of certain key vitamins and minerals is in severe decline.

Milk and the other dairy products provide:

- **Protein** On average milk provides 15 per cent of the protein in young people's diets and 12 per cent in those of adults. Milk is absolutely vital to vegetarians and semi-vegetarians.
- **Vitamin A – retinol** About 18 per cent comes from dairy products but today we consume only half to two-thirds the amount that was being consumed 15 years ago. Intake of fuller-fat dairy products is absolutely vital and should be higher.
- **Vitamin B2 – riboflavin** This is essential for energy release and is abundant in dairy products which provide 30 per cent of this vitamin. Approximately another 20 per cent comes from breakfast cereals, especially fortified varieties, so a quality milk and cereal breakfast is essential for the supply of riboflavin.
- **Calcium** About 50 per cent of all the calcium intake in the UK comes from milk, and poor intake in the growing years adds greatly to the risk of osteoporosis in later life.
- **Iodine** About 50 per cent of this trace element, which is necessary for thyroid function and metabolism comes from dairy products.
- **Energy** In the form of fats and sugar as well as protein.

*

It is not hard to realise that you will soon be in trouble if you do not consume much in the way of dairy products unless you also eat a very good diet. This would have to contain soya and soya milk, nuts and seeds, fish and possibly some liver or a vitamin supplement (for vitamin A). The decline in vitamin A intake over the last 15 years is very worrying as the average amount is now below the recommended figure. Outright deficiency is rare but reduced resistance to infection, particularly urinary and chest infections, are known problems associated with vitamin A deficiency. Fully skimmed milk contains virtually no vitamin A, while full milk and semi-skimmed are rich sources. The very low fat yoghurts are also unlikely to contain much vitamin A, although low fat hard cheese is still very nutritious.

As a rough guide we would be better off nutritionally to increase our dairy consumption by about 50 per cent and avoid the very low fat versions of milk and yoghurt.

Who isn't getting enough?
- Anyone consuming less than one litre of milk per week.
- Anyone who only consumes fully skimmed milk and very low fat, or virtually fat-free yoghurt and low fat cottage cheese, as in the process of removing all the fat, all the fat-soluble vitamin A is lost. This now poses a real danger of causing deficiency of this vitamin in a way not seen in Europe since the end of the First World War!
- Anyone on a dairy-free diet, unless they are consuming two litres of soya milk with added calcium and vitamin A.
- High consumers of fizzy drinks, which not only switch off the appetite for milk, but also have a high phosphoric acid content which further damages the balance of calcium.
- Regular or heavy drinkers of alcohol. These people almost never consume much in the way of dairy products and the alcohol damages the balance of calcium and vitamin B.
- Anyone with deficiencies of vitamin A, riboflavin and iodine.

What you can do about it
- Copy your parents or grandparents!

- Drink at least one and preferably two litres of full-fat or semi-skimmed milk (but not fully skimmed milk) per week. This can be consumed as milk shakes, hot chocolate, milk on your cereal at breakfast or as a snack in the evening. It doesn't matter how you do it, but do try to have milk instead of cola or fizz.
- If you are allergic or intolerant of cows' milk drink soya milk with added calcium and vitamin A.
- Eat about 112–125g of cheese per week. Lower fat Cheddar and Edam are very good for you, but avoid low-fat cottage cheese.
- Don't bother with the 'virtually fat-free' yoghurts or desserts unless they actually state that they have decent vitamin A content. I have yet to see one.
- Have butter if you so wish. Butter provides lots of retinol (vitamin A), so too does margarine, as it is fortified by law. There needs to be a similar law for fully skimmed milk as well!
- Have cream or ice-cream if you like provided you are not overweight. Put it with something healthy such as fresh fruit.
- Don't worry about fat. Many people will be better off having dairy products with a modest amount of fat and to reducing calorie energy intake by cutting back on sugar and alcohol, while at the same time increasing the amount of exercise they take.

Fresh fruit and vegetables
Why we need them
Numerous studies have looked at who eats which foods and who suffers from which diseases. Virtually all of these studies agree that regularly eating fruit and vegetables helps to:
- protect you from heart disease
- lower the risk of many types of cancer including bowel cancer, cervical cancer and to a lesser extent breast cancer
- lower the risk of diabetes in later life especially if you eat salad

- provide essential vitamins, especially vitamin C and folate
- provide essential minerals, especially potassium and magnesium
- provide fibre which helps with bowel regularity and lowers the risk of appendicitis and gall stones
- may help with hormonally-related problems, especially premenstrual syndrome.

How much do we need?

Once the importance of fresh fruit and vegetables to health and longevity was realised the scientific community, after much debate, came up with a simple target for us all to achieve – five, yes FIVE portions of fruit and vegetables per day. These should include some green vegetables and some yellow/orange fruits or vegetables. This will give us a good spread of vitamins and minerals as well as fibre. Basically the scientists came up with the kind of advice that our parent or grandparent would have given us.

To achieve this you will need to consume 35 servings of fruit and vegetables per week. Young adolescents will need fewer but three to four servings per day is a reasonable target for them. Thirty-five portions of fruit and vegetables will fill two shopping bags and should be purchased over two or three shopping trips per week, as the shelf-life of the nutrients is relatively short.

How much do we eat?

On average adults in the UK eat a total of 461g of fresh fruit and 42g of tinned fruit per week. One apple weighs approximately 120g which is equal to only four portions per week! Fresh vegetable consumption is better and works out at about seven portions per week. Salad foods, including raw carrots and tomatoes, both raw and cooked, come in at two to three portions of good size. So on average adults consume only half the amount that experts recommend.

We do like our potatoes as we put away 882g per week, about half of them as chips or roast potatoes. This is the equivalent of one small portion per day. Fresh potatoes, even as chips, are an important source of vitamin C in the British diet. Convenience forms are not so nutritious.

Unfortunately there is a marked difference in consumption with age. Adults over the age of 50 eat almost twice as much fruit and green leafy vegetables as those aged below 24. The under 24 year olds however do eat more peas, mainly frozen, and baked beans than their parents. These are actually quite nutritious and many young people would be less well nourished if they did not eat them.

Looking more closely at the lower consumption by those aged 15 to 18 years there is even more cause for concern. Vegetables, it would appear, are also poisonous to this age group. Young adults eat only about half as many fruit and vegetables as their parents, who only eat about half the recommended intake! This very low intake of fruit and vegetables explains many of the poor results of vitamin and mineral intake, especially of folic acid and magnesium.

Who is at risk of fruit and vegetable deficiency?

- all young men and women unless they are in a home where the parents are regular high fruit and vegetable consumers, for example, if their parents are greengrocers, farmers, dietitians or write books on nutrition!
- anyone living alone
- young people living away from home for the first time
- anyone who buys food once per week or less
- anyone living in an institution, for example nurses or those at boarding school
- anyone with symptoms of vitamin C and B deficiency
- anyone with a lack of fibre in their diet – who isn't able to open their bowels most days without difficulty
- there is a slight increased risk if you live in Scotland or the north of England or are less well off, but these factors are small.

Many of us do not make the target, and you may well ask why. Well, when did you last see cabbage advertised on TV?

Health effects of fruit and vegetable deficiency

As well as the increased risks of heart disease, diabetes and cancer there are a whole host of health problems that are more likely to occur if you don't eat enough fruit and vegetables:

- premenstrual syndrome and period problems
- constipation
- depression if due to poor vitamin and mineral balance
- muscle pains if due to potassium and magnesium deficiency
- fatigue if due to vitamin and mineral deficiency
- kidney stones
- appendicitis.

It's your choice. Just making a little effort with your diet and increasing your fruit and vegetable consumption can save you an awful lot of health trouble now and in the longer term.

What can you do about it?

Remember you are aiming to double your intake of fruit and vegetables.

- Make a list of all the fruits and vegetables that you actually like.
- Go shopping for fresh fruit and vegetables at least twice a week and buy plenty. Be adventurous and buy some different vegetables or exotic fruits.
- Always keep fresh carrots, tomatoes, peppers and cucumber in your fridge, and frozen peas, tinned beans and sweetcorn as stand-by foods.
- If you have a good canteen at work have your main meal there and eat less pasta, fewer potatoes and more vegetables.
- If you are busy at work, buy a ready prepared bag of salad for your evening meal on your way home. It may be expensive, but it is both convenient and nutritious.
- Don't be lazy. Vegetables take a bit of effort but not much, and don't be afraid to get your hands dirty peeling them.
- Take fruit to work or have some in your car.

- Keep a bowl of fruit in your home, preferably as close to the TV as possible.
- At the end of each day, or as you decide what to have for dinner, ask yourself the question 'Did I eat FIVE?'

Tea, coffee and caffeine

Why do we need then?

We don't, but we do like them. Britain was once regarded as a nation of tea-drinkers. It's till true but coffee consumption is beginning to rival that of tea.

Before I deal with the possible harmful effects of tea, coffee, cola and chocolate let me say a few kind words about their benefits, as nothing is all bad. These beverages are refreshing because they contain caffeine and related compounds that act as mild stimulants, which help us to combat fatigue and may improve alertness. Caffeine also improves the effect of painkillers and acts as a mild diuretic. Instant coffee contains 150mg per mug, filter coffee about 250mg per mug, and tea about 100mg per mug. Doses of 250mg will produce a noticeable effect in many people, so more than two or three cups can produce a variety of undesirable effects. Women are much more sensitive to caffeine than men, as are non-smokers, and these two groups, as well as pregnant women, typically consume fewer caffeinated beverages.

Tea is made from the dried leaves of Indian and Chinese tea plants. The young leaves are rich in folate, some of the other B vitamins and the trace element manganese. Tea provides some 5 per cent or more of the folate in our diet. Tea can also slow down the passage of food through the gut and is helpful in the recovery from gastroenteritis.

Coffee has the opposite effect, stimulating the bowel, and can act as a mild laxative. It has no significant nutritional content.

Chocolate has a good content of potassium, a little protein and quite a lot of fat. When eaten in the form of a chocolate bar it comes with a high content of sugar but as a chocolate drink the added milk adds plenty of calcium and protein.

Cola has nothing in its favour when compared with a glass of water.

The undesirable health effects of tea and coffee
Too much caffeine causes a number of mild but sometimes more troublesome adverse effects including:
- palpitations
- anxiety and premenstrual syndrome
- increased urination
- insomnia – delay in getting to sleep
- tremors of the hands
- migraine headaches.

Apart from the effects of caffeine too much tea and coffee can have other effects too:
- constipation from tea
- diarrhoea from coffee
- indigestion and heartburn from coffee and possibly tea
- blocking the absorption of iron from vegetarian foods due to the tannin in tea – this is a very important factor in contributing to mild iron deficiency in vegetarian women
- reduced absorption of magnesium and possibly other minerals from coffee, probably because of shortening the time for food to be digested and absorbed.

What can you do about it?
Aim for a safe intake. It is wise to cut down if you have any of the above health problems but do so gradually over two or three weeks otherwise a withdrawal headache, which may turn into a migraine, can develop. It is best not to drink any tea or coffee after 5pm as it can take about six hours for caffeine to clear out of your system.

A safe daily intake is:
- one mug or two small cups of coffee
- two cups of tea
- an occasional can of a fizzy drink, for example cola – one

per week (see Fizzy drinks and squash on page 36)
- young people, pregnant women and those with a tendency to anxiety or insomnia are better to have none.

Good alternatives are:
- Rooibos or redbush tea, which is a natural tea 'look-alike' when made with milk and contains no caffeine and very little tannin
- herb and fruit teas
- decaffeinated versions of tea and coffee
- fizzy mineral water with a little fruit juice or a squeeze of lemon
- fruit juices
- water and milk and fortified soya milk, which are the best drinks for young growing people who wish to be healthy.

Salt
Why do we need it?
We need some sodium salt but nowhere near as much as we actually consume. Sodium or salt deficiency is exceptionally rare and hardly ever occurs as a result of dietary inadequacy.

Our bodies retain sodium in solution in the blood and in the fluid that surrounds all the cells of the body. It is needed to maintain the electrical activity of cells, particularly in the nervous system and muscles. The kidney has the task of excreting any excess salt, which is inevitable if you eat a Western diet. The problem most encountered is too much rather than too little sodium salt.

How much do we consume?
About 15 per cent of our intake comes coming from table salt added to cooking or at the table and 85 per cent from hidden sources in pre-prepared foods. The biggest food sources of salt are bread, cheese and salted butter, bacon, sausages and other preserved meats, savoury snacks such as crisps and nuts, many

tinned foods such as baked beans, tomato ketchup and pickled foods.

On average men consume about 3.5g and women 2.5g per day so the minimum requirement of 0.5g is achieved by all. The upper safe amount is considered by some experts to be in the region of 3.5g which would mean that about half of all men and approximately 10 per cent of all women eat too much salt. Fifteen to 18-year-olds consume more than this. They eat more white bread, breakfast cereals, pizza, crisps and other savoury snacks, bacon and sausages, and these are the foods most heavily advertised. Alas, they barely contain a desirable mineral or essential vitamin between them, just plenty of 'empty calories'.

Health effects of excess salt

Not everyone who eats too much sodium salt really has a problem. If you have one or more of the problems below then you will probably need to cut down on your intake:

- High blood pressure – about one-third of those with a high blood pressure will experience a small but significant drop in their blood pressure if they cut back on salt and salty foods.
- Those with a family history of high blood pressure. The effect of salt is often determined by a family tendency and it is never too early to cut back.
- Fluid retention. Water retention is only possible if the diet is high in sodium. Ankle swelling, finger swelling and abdominal bloating, especially if they are worse premenstrually, can all be due to too much sodium in the diet. You will need to cut down, possibly very strictly, to achieve a good result.
- Kidney stones. These are most often due to an excess of calcium being lost in the urine. This appears to happen when the intake of sodium is high.
- Osteoporosis is also due to the silent departure of calcium from the body, much of it in the urine. So if you are at increased risk, as many of us are, then cut back on sodium.

- Magnesium and potassium deficiency, as the balance of these minerals may be worsened by a high sodium intake.

Who is at risk of excess salt?
- virtually everyone to some degree
- those with premenstrual syndrome where fluid retention is a problem
- Many young people with a low intake of fresh fruit and vegetables, who are at risk of deficiencies in magnesium and potassium
- All of those with high blood pressure, fluid retention, kidney stones and osteoporosis.

What you can do about it
- Cut down, cut down, cut down. For many a realistic goal is to halve salt intake. Do this by cutting out or cutting back on those foods that are high in salt and are low in essential nutrients. Bread and cheese are quite high in salt but are very nutritious so they should not be the first things to go.
- Avoid adding salt to the cooking or at the table. At least taste your food first before you add any. You won't miss the taste of salt so much if you use more herbs and spices.
- Cut right back on salty snacks such as crisps and salted nuts. A small packet once or twice a week is the maximum that should be allowed.
- Limit or avoid any convenience meals such as pizza, prepared meals and cooked meats all of which are high in salt. Fresh home-made meals are a lot lower in sodium.
- Limit the consumption of bacon and sausages to once or twice per week.
- Limit bread to three or four slices per day and cheese to 120–175g per week.
- Eat out less often. Most fast-food and meals served in restaurants are quite heavily salted.
- If you have to have salt use low sodium substitute, like LoSalt but use sparingly as they still contain about one-third of the sodium when compared to normal salt. Some

manufacturers are now using a type of combined sodium/potassium salt in manufactured foods which is a great improvement.

- Persevere. It takes about six weeks for your taste buds to adjust to a reduced salt diet but it is worth it. Once you have made the change you will soon recognise when food is poor quality and over-salted.

Alcohol

Alcohol has become increasingly popular over the last 50 years and total consumption has doubled in that time. We drink more and differently, and this is not without effects upon our health.

In the past alcohol, particularly in the form of beer or ale, was the deserved drink of working men who would consume one or many pints during the evening not only to relax, but to return the fluid lost from a hard day's labour and to give them the energy for the next. Nowadays we do not labour as people did a century ago, yet many of us feel we need a glass or two of wine each night to help us relax after a day's work, or several cocktails or designer beers at the weekend in order to enjoy ourselves. What can be wrong with that? Well not much if it is in moderation. A safe modest allowance is up to 14 units per week for men and up to 21 units for men, and not all in one go! A more careful level allowance is up to 10 units, equal to about a bottle of wine, per week and less, about two or three drinks per week, for those who are trying to get pregnant. Drinking two or three glasses of wine per day may help to reduce the risk of heart disease in some middle-aged men but this is no reason for you to drink so much.

Measuring alcohol

Doctors and nutritionists measure alcohol in units. A unit is 10 ml of alcohol – about 8g. A bottle of wine of 750ml is usually 12 per cent alcohol. This is equal to 90ml which is nine units. So a small glass of wine which is one-sixth of a bottle is one-and-a-half units. Beer and lagers are getting stronger and stronger as it seems we want more alcohol in a smaller volume of fluid and fewer calories per drink so that we can drink more!

Too much alcohol

The problems with too much alcohol consumption are threefold:

- It provides lots of empty calories.
- It knocks out many vitamins and minerals.
- It has many diverse undesirable health effects.

Empty calories

Each unit of alcohol contains 8g of alcohol which alone will provide 32 calories. But most alcohol, except for spirits, will come with a variety of sugars and flavourings which in turn will provide many more calories. The calorie content of alcohol is not low, so apart from the health drawbacks, there are weight-gain implications for everyone other than those in the skinny brigade.

The calories you can expect to find in a typical glass of your favourite drinks is as follows:

- White wine (medium)   75 calories per 100ml glass
- Red wine   68 calories per 100 ml glass
- Spirits (gin, vodka, brandy etc)   55 calories per shot
- Lager   65 calories per 225ml glass (½ pint)
- Beer (draught)   72 calories per 225ml glass (½ pint)

The nutrient content of most alcoholic drinks is minimal. They contain no protein and tiny amounts of minerals and vitamins. The one main exception is beer which contains modest amounts of magnesium and small amounts of vitamin B. But don't get excited because in order to metabolise the alcohol you are going to need a lot more vitamin B and magnesium than any beer can provide. So the more you drink the more deficient you are likely to become.

Unfortunately most of us who drink too much have done little or nothing to 'earn' our drink in terms of energy requirement. This means that the more we drink the fatter we get, or the less of other good food we eat. Alcohol thus has a displacing effect upon the other desirable components of our diet such as protein and quality carbohydrate, which are major providers of those ever important vitamins and minerals.

Health effects of alcohol

Immediate:
- facial flushing – and may worsen many facial skin problems
- depression
- obesity
- higher blood pressure
- migraine headaches
- increases the chances of accidents of all types
- fatigue
- low blood sugar and dips in energy level
- period problems
- problems during pregnancy, including poor growth of the baby.

Delayed effects include the increased risk of many health problems such as:
- cancer, including breast cancer
- high blood pressure and stroke
- liver disease
- damage to the nervous system
- heart problems
- osteoporosis
- many nutrition-related problems.

The effect of alcohol on vitamins and minerals

Too much alcohol will adversely effect the balance of just about every vitamin and mineral that you can think of, but some are especially vulnerable.
- *Vitamin B1 Thiamin* can become severely deficient from

alcohol excess especially if there is associated vomiting. Loss of short-term memory is a classic feature of this deficiency, which if prolonged becomes permanent.

- *Folic acid* is another of the B vitamins vital during pregnancy which if deficient, results in depression. Deficiency is more likely in those who drink heavily. All the other B vitamins are also damaged by too much alcohol, with other effects upon mood, concentration and digestion.
- *Calcium* is not provided by alcoholic drinks and above average alcohol intake is a risk factor for osteoporosis.
- *Magnesium* is also flushed out by the booze and will lead to muscle cramps and depressed mood.
- *Zinc* too can become severely deficient and this is likely to influence resistance to infection.
- Finally, because of the 'displacement effect' of alcoholic drinks, the overall intake of many other minerals as well as vitamins and essential fatty acids is likely to be reduced.

Fizzy drinks & squash

These have become popular over the last 30 years and have, to a large degree, replaced tap water and milk as the most popular drinks of the young. 'What's wrong with them?' I hear you cry. Nothing of course in moderation, but we passed moderate consumption levels over 20 years ago. Now there's no stopping us. In the mid-1980s the average adult consumption of fizzy drinks was about one litre per week, equivalent to three 330ml cans or two 500ml bottles. Teenage girls now consume 1.3 litres per week and boys over 1.8 litres per week of which about one third are low-calorie varieties. What is worrying is that within the teenage population there are some very high consumers who will drink one or two cans each day, consuming 3 litres or more per week.

Each litre of carbonated drink such as cola provides:
- 410 calories, excess of which will turn to fat
- 150mg of the mineral phosphate which has to be balanced with calcium in the diet

- approximately 138mg of caffeine which acts as a stimulant.

Health effects of fizzy drinks and squash

- Too many calories from the huge amount of sugar (equivalent to seven teaspoons per 330ml can).
- Too much caffeine which will act as a stimulant and worsen:
    anxiety
    insomnia
    migraine headaches.
- Too much Phosphate mineral which will unbalance calcium causing:
    Lowered blood calcium
    Increased risk of muscle cramps, and possibly epilepsy.

A safe limit is probably two 330 ml cans per week, which is less than half current consumption levels.

CHAPTER 4

Designing your health plan

For 18 years I have been designing plans for individuals in order to help them feel healthy and look good. Now, through the pages of *The Model Plan*, you have the opportunity to use the wealth of experience to write your own tailor-made health plan. Between us we need to tailor your programme to suit your individual requirements; this involves taking into consideration your tastes, your lifestyle, your budget and of course the needs of your body.

As you read through the chapters that follow you will come across recommendations that are just right for your situation. Rather than relying on your memory, I would like you to make a note of them on the Healthy Eating Plan, which you will find at the end of this chapter. Gradually your list of notes will turn into your own personal health plan, which you can then follow during the next few months.

Before getting started with the plan, let's consider some of the key issues.

Your tastes

However your dietary recommendations turn out, they must appeal to you. There is absolutely no point in trying to force yourself to swallow food that you dislike, no matter how healthy it may be. There are always good alternatives, so if you don't like something, the rule is, 'Don't include it'.

Your budget

The diet and supplement plan you design must fit in with your budget. There is no point planning to buy expensive options if you are living on a student budget or are unemployed. Realistically, it will cost somewhere between £30 and £35 to eat well each week, including lunch. It is possible to cut the cost down a bit by eating more vegetarian options, as these are usually cheaper than meat and fish.

Sometimes it helps to review the whole of our budget, and perhaps deploy some funds from elsewhere to the food kitty. Very often, when you start looking closely, you may find that quite a bit of money is being spent on chocolate, or cigarettes and alcohol, or perhaps on entertainment and clothes. One survey we did a few years ago showed that people were spending between £5 and £15 per week on chocolate and junk food!

Your lifestyle

It is important to consider your lifestyle when composing your plan. For example, if you go out to the gym or to work in the evening, straight from your day job or your studies, it is unlikely that you will be home to eat dinner at the usual time, so you may need a wholesome snack to tide you over. Working shifts will mean that you need to make a special plan, so that you still get your three proper meals each day with a few wholesome snacks thrown in. If you spend your day in an isolated area, and the only food available at lunch time is sandwiches, maybe you need to consider organising lunch at home the night before and taking it with you.

Whatever you do it is important to eat wholesome food, little and often. Never miss a meal, as your blood sugar levels will drop, and you will be tempted to go back to your old habits. Besides, your body actually needs a constant supply of good nutrients in order to function properly.

Meeting your needs

At the end of each chapter in Part Two you will find a list of recommendations to follow. Some will involve making significant dietary changes, at least in the short-term. Initially this may involve cutting out certain common foods and concentrating on eating some more specialised foods. If you are the shopper and the cook this will work well, but if not you will need to make a plan. If you live at home with your family, or with a friend or partner, and you eat together, you will need to make them familiar with your new plan. If someone else does the cooking, take time to sit with them and explain, showing them the suggested menu plans you will be following and any relevant recipes. Having the support of those around you while you are following your plan will help enormously.

Don't like cooking!

As few of us have had any formal cookery lessons, it may be that you are not used to cooking and would therefore prefer not to. The Healthy Eating Plan was written with you in mind. It is simple and easy to follow, and does not require a great deal in the way of cookery skills. There are plenty of fast options that often do not require any cooking at all, and yet they do deliver the goodies in terms of nutrients.

There are lots of short-cuts available these days. For example, if you would like to eat chicken, but don't want to cook it, you can buy it ready cooked. The same goes for soup. Home-made soup is delicious, but fewer and fewer of us have the time to stand over the cooker on a regular basis. There are a variety of 'home-made' type soups available in supermarkets made with wholesome ingredients.

Addressing your problems

Whether it is acne, PMS or your energy levels that you need to target, you will be able to incorporate the recommendations into your health plan. As you go through each section, note down the relevant recommendations on your plan. By the time you have finished, you will have a complete list of dietary recommendations, a list of supplement recommendations, if they apply, and you will have devised a workable exercise routine to follow that fits in with your lifestyle.

Wholesome and tasty

Whether you choose to follow the Healthy Eating Plan, which begins on page 158 or have a go at the Discovery Diet, which you will find on page 172, you can feel confident that you will be getting all the nutrients you need in order to flourish. There are plenty of options to choose from, which allows you the flexibility to design the plan according to your tastes.

If you are a vegetarian, or would like to follow the vegetarian diet, there is the opportunity to use the vegetarian menus, which begin on page 167. A good vegetarian diet can deliver the nutrients you need, but all too often those following a vegetarian regime are not sufficiently educated about how to balance their diet. There are degrees of vegetarianism – for example those who consume dairy products as well as vegetables and vegetarian protein are known as lacto-vegetarian, and those who consume eggs as well as dairy products are known as ovo-lacto-vegetarian. Vegans are more strict and only consume vegetable derived foods. These days, there are growing numbers of people who prefer not to eat meat, but are still happy to include fish in their diets.

A major problem with vegetarian and vegan diets is that they may contain a borderline or poor quality protein intake. Protein-rich vegetarian foods include nuts, seeds, peas, beans, lentils, whole grains, brown rice, sprouted beans and soya bean products, which need to be combined in order to provide the body with all the amino acids it would normally derive from meat or fish.

Enjoy your food

Use the section Good Food – Where to Find It on page 307 to hunt down the foods that you enjoy. There are ever-increasing numbers of tasty new products on the market these days so make sure you look out for them. There is a wide variety of products on the list, so don't be afraid to experiment. Our tastes differ enormously, so don't expect to like everything you try!

Don't forget to make a shopping list before you go out to shop for food, and never go shopping on an empty stomach!

Healthy Eating Plan

A. Dietary Recommendations

Tick which option you will be following: ✔

1. Healthy Eating Plan ◯   2. Discovery Diet ◯

B. Special Rules

1. ....

2. ....

3. ....

4. ....

5. ....

6. ....

7. ....

8. ....

9. ....

10. ....

C. Supplements
   1. . . . .
   2. . . . .
   3. . . . .
   4. . . . .

D. Exercise
   . . . .
   . . . .
   . . . .
   . . . .

E. Other recommendations
   . . . .
   . . . .
   . . . .
   . . . .

F. Things to ask my doctor
   . . . .
   . . . .
   . . . .
   . . . .

G. Additional notes
   . . . .
   . . . .
   . . . .
   . . . .

CHAPTER 5

Is diet enough?

Whether we can get enough nutrients from our diet alone is a controversial question. The scientific camps remain divided, as some experts believe we can while other respected authorities do not.

If you scored 18 or above on the questionnaire 'Is Your Diet Good For You?' on page 12, then the chances are you are getting lots of nutrients from your diet. However, if your score was lower, you may need to consider taking some supplements, particularly in the short-term, while you make improvements to your diet and allow time for them to take effect.

Before making any big decisions one way or the other, complete this questionnaire, which will enable you to assess the nutrient levels in your body.

Are you in good nutritional shape?

Tick yes or no against each sign or symptom.

Fatigue   yes ○   **no** ○

Significance   Anaemia, mixed vitamin B or magnesium deficiencies, also under-active thyroid and other problems

Action   See your doctor for blood tests including vitamin B12 if vegan or vegetarian, and consider a strong multivitamin and mineral supplement.

Pale appearance   yes ○ no ○
Significance   Anaemia – iron, folate or vitamin B12 deficiencies
Action   See your doctor for appropriate tests.

Heavy periods with flooding or clots   yes ○ no ○
Significance   Iron deficiency
Action   See your doctor for tests including serum ferritin. Take
                    supplements of iron or iron and multivitamins.

Painful periods needing painkillers   yes ○ no ○
Significance   Possible magnesium deficiency
Action   Consider taking magnesium supplements 150–300mg
                    per day and evening primrose oil and fish oil.

Irregular periods   yes ○ no ○
Significance   Underweight, low protein diet and excess alcohol
Action   Better diet and strong multivitamin preparation.

Recurrent mouth ulcers or sore smooth tongue   yes ○ no ○
Significance   Iron, folate and vitamin B12
Action   See your doctor for the appropriate tests. Consider
                    taking multivitamin and iron supplement.

Sore bleeding gums   yes ○ no ○
Significance   Vitamin C
Action   Take 1000mg Vitamin C with bioflavanoids per day
                    and visit your dental hygienist.

Excessive cracking and peeling of the lips   yes ○ no ○
Significance   Vitamin B2 – riboflavin
Action   Consider taking a strong vitamin B preparation.

Cracking at the corners of the eyes   yes ○ no ○
Significance   Vitamin B2 and vitamin B6
Action   Consider taking a strong multivitamin and mineral
                    preparation.

Cracking at the corners of the mouth   yes ○ no ○
Significance   Iron, and/or mixed vitamin B deficiency. Thrush and
                    eczema also possible.
Action   Multivitamin with iron, see your doctor if it persists.

Red greasy skin at the sides of the nose   yes ○ no ○
Significance   Vitamin B2 – Riboflavin and/or vitamin B6 deficiency
                    and/or zinc.
Action   Strong B complex supplement, and 15mg of zinc per day.

Combination skin   yes ○ no ○
Significance   Mixed vitamin B and/or zinc
Action   Strong B complex supplement, and 15mg of zinc per
                 day.

Persistant dandruff   yes ○ no ○
Significance   Biotin and essential fatty acid deficiency
Action   Multivitamins, biotin 500mcgs and high-strength fish
                 oils. Also, antifungal, tea-tree or tar-based shampoos.

Eczema   yes ○ no ○
Significance   Possible Omega 6 essential fatty acid deficiency if
                 excessive dryness
Action   Evening primrose oil 3,000mg per day. See doctor for
                 allergy assessment and infection inspection.

Red scaly skin in sun exposed areas   yes ○ no ○
Significance   Vitamin B3 – nicotinamide deficiency
Action   Strong vitamin B with 100mg of Nicotinamide

Acne   yes ○ no ○
Significance   Possible zinc deficiency
Action   Zinc supplement 15 mg per day (30 mg if supervised).

Psoriasis   yes ○ no ○
Significance   Possible mixed vitamin B, zinc and essential fatty acid
                 deficiencies
Action   Strong multivitamin, zinc 15mg and high-strength fish
                 oil supplements. Combine with conventional treatment.

Excessively dry skin   yes ○ no ○
Significance   Possible mixed deficiency of essential fatty acids, vitamin
                 A and vitamin E
Action   Multivitamin and mineral supplement with evening
                 primrose oil 2,000g and high-strength fish oil, plus
                 400iu of vitamin E.

Rough red pimply skin on the upper arms and/or thighs yes ○ no ○
Significance   None if mild. If severe, mixed vitamin and essential fatty
                 acid deficiency
Action   Multivitamin and mineral supplement with evening
                 primrose oil 2,000g and high-strength fish oil and better
                 diet.

Depression, anxiety and premenstrual syndrome yes ○ no ○

Significance   Possible mixed vitamin B, and/or magnesium
                 deficiencies

Action   Magnesium-rich strong multivitamin and mineral
                 supplement with additional magnesium 150–300mg per
                 day.

Split, brittle or flattened or upturned nails yes ○ no ○

Significance   Iron deficiency

Action   Iron supplement. See your doctor if persistent.

Ridged nails and white spots on nails yes ○ no ○

Significance   Uncertain significance, possibly iron and zinc

Action   Better diet, and multivitamin and mineral supplement.

Poor hair growth or generalised thinning and loss of hair yes ○ no ○

Significance   Mild iron deficiency and vitamin C

Action   See your doctor for tests for anaemia including Serum
                 Ferritin and thyroid function. Take iron and
                 multivitamin supplements and 1000mg of Vitamin C.

Loss of sense of taste yes ○ no ○

Significance   Possible zinc deficiency

Action   Zinc 15mg per day (30 mg if under supervision). See
                 your doctor if it persists.

Poor vision at night or in the dark yes ○ no ○

Significance   Possible vitamin A (Retinol) and/or zinc deficiency

Action   Multivitamin and zinc supplement 15mg per day (30mg
                 if under supervision). You must see your doctor.

Poor appetite yes ○ no ○

Significance   Zinc, iron and/or mixed vitamin B deficiencies

Action   Multivitamin and multimineral supplement. See your
                 doctor if you have lost weight.

Wrinkles yes ○ no ○

Significance   Possible lack of antioxidants – Vitamins A,C,E, and the
                 minerals selenium and zinc

Action   Consider taking a good strong multivitamin and mineral
                 preparation.

Your score

• If you ticked **no** in 25 or more categories, you are a star.

The chances are you are in pretty good nutritional shape, and there will be no real need for you to take nutritional supplements, unless you particularly want to take a multivitamin and mineral supplement to protect yourself against the potentially harmful effects of the environment.

- A score of 20–24 negatives means that you are not doing too badly, but there are some issues that need addressing. Improving your diet and making it more nutrient-dense is the first action to take, and then consider taking the supplements recommended for your particular problems.

- If you ticked fewer than 20 **no's**, you will obviously need to take some supplement as well as making some fairly major changes to your diet. Follow the Healthy Eating Plan on page 158, and take the supplements recommended for your particular problems.

Which supplements?

In recent years the supplement industry has hit boom time. However, as there are so many varieties available, and they are often of varying quality, there is much confusion about what to take, and whether there is a real pay-back from a monthly investment.

There are times when supplements are really useful, as you can see from the questionnaire you have just completed, and it is worth bearing in mind that the longer you have experienced the signs and symptoms the more likely you are to have one or more nutritional deficiencies.

Here is a guide to making supplement choices. Most of them are available in chemists and health food shops, but some of the better quality, specialist brands are only available by mail order. Details of the WNAS can be found on page 317.

- **Ordinary multivitamins** There are many types to choose from. The better ones have a good range of vitamins and sometimes minerals at a level close to the RDA (recommended daily allowance), or RNI (recommended nutrient intake), and the likely cost is approximately 5–10p per day.

- **Multivitamins and iron** These are similar to those mentioned above, but contain additional iron, which is often needed by women with heavy or prolonged periods.
- **Strong multivitamins** These often contain 5–30 times the usual daily requirement of some of the B vitamins. Actually that is not a bad idea if your diet isn't utterly brilliant, especially if you like to drink alcohol, or if you experience anxiety or depression. Some may help with particular problems. Optivite, for example, is a magnesium-rich supplement for women, which has been through four successful clinical trials for premenstrual syndrome. Unfortunately these days it is only available by mail order.
- **Mineral supplements** There are a wide variety available: iron for heavy periods, zinc to help with acne and poor healing, calcium to help prevent the bone thinning disease osteoporosis – though this is best combined with exercise and magnesium. Magnesium can also be used as a laxative, can help premenstrual problems and period pains and may benefit some types of fatigue.

Case History

Rachel, who was only 19 years old, had been given a diagnosis of chronic fatigue by her GP and hospital specialist a few months before she came to the clinic.

A year earlier she had had a severe bout of gastric 'flu after which she became increasingly tired. At her worst she slept 20 hours per day, was losing weight, had muscle pains, fatigue and recurrent mouth ulcers. All the tests at the hospital had been normal except, she said, for a low vitamin B level. It turned out that she had been found to have a slightly low vitamin B12 level. This was nearly ignored but she was given three injections of vitamin B12 by the hospital. A series of tests to see why she was deficient followed and they did not reveal anything untoward. Her diet was quite adequate in vitamin B12 as she ate meat or fish several times per week. A possible explanation for her deficiency was that she was taking the oral contraceptive pill and this might have lowered her vitamin B12 level. Other tests revealed that she was also low in vitamin B1.

Following the vitamin B12 injections and after taking some strong supplements of vitamin B complex she made a full recovery. She returned to needing only eight hours sleep and after six months was able to go off trekking abroad for eight weeks. She stopped the pill and will have to take care if she takes it again.

Make a note of the following scientifically-based supplements as the supplement market tends to be crowded and confusing.

- *Calcium* Calcium carbonate, lactate or citrate is useful for anyone on a low calcium diet – for example, a dairy-free or a vegan diet. A typical dosage is 300–600mg daily. It can be taken as a preventative measure for a low calcium diet and is best taken with meals, but must not be taken with bran.
- *Magnesium* as oxide, citrate or chelate. Supplements provide 100–150mg per tablet. It is useful for premenstrual syndrome, muscle cramps or constipation. Higher doses act effectively as a laxative.
- *Vitamin C* at doses of between 2–4g per day, *zinc* at doses of 30mg per day and *vitamin A* as Palmitate at doses of 25,000 iu per day, can also help to boost the immune system if you are in a low state or suffering with a post viral condition.

It may well be worth trying a course of supplements to see how you get on. While vitamins and minerals can be taken in the long-term, the herbal preparations are usually best taken while addressing a particular problem. For example, a course of echinacea to boost the immune system will last for anything from a few weeks to a month, and the recommended course for St John's Wort to help with depression or Seasonal Affective Disorder (SAD) is three months. If you feel you need some extra help you can contact the WNAS for advice. The contact details are on page 317.

- *Evening primrose oil* This is helpful for eczema, premenstrual breast tenderness and period pain.
- *Marine fish oil* This is particularly good for helping skin problems like dry skin and psoriasis, as well as helpful with painful periods.
- *Folic acid* 400mcg of folic acid should be taken by women who are trying to conceive, or who may fall pregnant, and it should be taken daily before conception through to the end of the first four months of pregnancy. It has been shown to reduce the risk of birth defects like spina bifida by as much as 70 per cent.
- *Antioxidants* Vitamin A (as betacarotene), natural vitamin E, and vitamin C (with bioflavenoids), and the minerals selenium, zinc, manganese and copper, help to protect us against cancer and environmental toxins.

Herbal Preparations A number of herbal preparations have been shown by clinical trials to be just as effective as drugs in helping to overcome certain symptoms.
- *St John's Wort* 'The sunshine supplement' – has been repeatedly shown to help overcome depression and is more widely prescribed by doctors in Germany than Prozac.
- *Echinacea* A herb that is used to boost the immune system.
- *Valerian* Helps to combat nervous tension and insomnia.
- *Feverfew and ginger* Help to prevent and reduce headaches.
- *Passiflora* Helps with anxiety, tension, irritability and sleeplessness.
- *Buchu* Helps to relieve wind and bloating.
- *Artichoke and slippery elm* Help to combat indigestion and soothes the gut.
- *Blue flag* Helps with acne, boils and other skin infections.
- *Primula* Helps to combat catarrh.
- *Black cohosh* Can help to relieve menstrual cramps.

CHAPTER 6

The feel-good factor

If you wake up feeling sluggish or a bit down, what can you do to send your spirits soaring within an hour?

- Discover you have won the lottery? That's doubtful.
- Get whisked off your feet by a dream partner? Unlikely first thing in the morning unless you have already identified the individual.
- Discover that all public transport is on strike for the day, so you can have a day off? Probably more realistic, but still unlikely.
- Spend the time dancing yourself into a sweat and singing your heart out to your favourite music? Not only likely, but realistic and possible.

Exercise to the point of breathlessness, apart from vigorous sex, or for some people, shopping, is one of the few pastimes that will influence your mood, hormone function and energy levels positively. Exercise is not just a nice idea as it is necessary for the optimum function, structure and preservation of muscles, bones, joints, and the heart. Not only does exercise give us the feel-good factor on the day, but it can also improve the quality of and extend active life. Regular exercise helps to prevent the debilitating and often fatal conditions of heart disease and stroke, and helps to prevent the crippling bone-thinning disease osteoporosis, which doesn't affect only older people. Research of the last few years shows that our bone mass reaches its peak by the time we reach our mid-twenties. It is therefore important to take regular weight-bearing exercise, in other words anything that involves impact between the floor and your feet, and to eat a wholesome diet in order to keep your bones in good condition.

In addition to these wonderful health benefits of exercise, it helps to keep our skin looking healthy as it promotes circulation. Also, the increased energy expenditure of exercise has a direct relationship to the amount of weight an overweight person is likely to lose, and the amount of food someone who is happy with their weight can eat without gaining additional kilos. For although obesity is associated with a raised blood cholesterol, heart disease, and high blood pressure, vigorous exercise reduces the risk of someone overweight contracting one of these conditions to almost the same level as someone of optimum weight for their height.

Exercise and weight loss

The energy used in the process of exercising burns additional calories and therefore helps to increase your resting metabolic rate. Providing you stick to the diet suggested, and don't consume lots of additional calories, you get into what is known as calorie deficit. This means that if you do an hour's vigorous exercise instead of sitting in a chair for an hour, you could burn up an extra 100–200 calories, which would otherwise have contributed to your waistline.

How much is enough?

I encourage people to exercise to the point of breathlessness in order to increase output from the heart, and trigger the release of the brain chemicals known as endorphins. While a regular exerciser may need to do a full hour of vigorous exercise in order to achieve this, a non-exerciser may only need to do a few minutes initially, until they have built up their stamina. Physical exercise is an important factor in maintaining fitness and energy balance, but you do need to begin exercising at the correct pace. If the exercise programme you choose is too vigorous at first, it will only leave you feeling achy, tired and disappointed. If, on the other hand, your exercises are insufficient to stimulate your limb and heart muscles, thus providing aerobic exercise, then you will effectively be wasting your time.

Must it be aerobics?

Many of us associate aerobic exercise with the local gym or an hour's workout, and while these activities will achieve increased cardiac output, there are other activities that will do the same job. Aerobic exercise is exercise that stimulates the large groups of muscles in your body, getting them to contract rhythmically. Over a period of time, these muscles, including the heart, which is a muscular organ, become more efficient. Eventually the heart in particular can work more slowly, but with increased capability. Once you have achieved increased cardiac function, you will usually experience an increased sense of well-being, both physically and mentally. Instead of feeling sluggish, you will feel energised and happy – you may even find yourself walking around singing out loud.

In order to protect your health, and to reap the ongoing benefits that aerobic exercise can provide, you must continue to exercise regularly, ideally for at least 30 to 40 minutes, four or five times per week. Apart from aerobics classes or gym workouts, there are many other forms of exercise from which you can choose. The bottom line is that it must be exercise that you enjoy, otherwise you won't stick to it for long. You can swim, jog, power-walk, skip, play racquet sports, cycle or even dance.

Choosing an exercise plan

Unless you are an established exerciser, ex̶ of breathlessness at least four times per ̶ answer the following exercise questionnaire.

Exercise Questionnaire

Tick any answer that applies to you now

Are you very overweight? (see page 56 for weight chart) ◯
Are you moderately overweight? ◯
Are you slightly overweight? ◯
Are you currently doing no exercise whatsoever? ◯
Are you currently doing some gentle exercise occasionally? ◯
Do you exercise once or twice per week in a formal setting? ◯
Do you exercise more than three times per week for more than half an hour each time? ◯
Do you get puffed out easily? ◯
Do you run up and down the stairs without panting? ◯
Which of the following best describes you?
- *Very unfit* ◯
- *Moderately unfit* ◯
- *Not as fit as you should be* ◯
- *Moderately fit* ◯
- *Fit* ◯
- *In excellent physical condition!* ◯

The graph on page 56 gives measurements for height and weight. It is divided up into five sections – 1, 0, 1, 2, and 3. These are grades of obesity based on weight and height taken from the formula originally devised by a Belgian scientist, Quetelet. Quetelet's Index, which is more usually known as Body Mass Index (BMI) – is widely used in the assessment of obesity. The formula is derived by multiplying the height by itself and dividing by the weight. Let's use mine as an example. I am 1.65m tall, so multiplied by itself that equals 2.72, then I divide my weight, which is 55.5K by 2.72 and get the result of 20.4. Unless your are brilliant at arithmetic you will need to

...ator, When you have your result you can check it
...t the categories below:

Grade -1:   less than 20
Grade 0:   20–25
Grade 1:   25–30
Grade 2:   30–40
Grade 3:   greater than 40

Normal or ideal weight is grade 0. Grade 1 is overweight, usually between 10 and 20 per cent above the ideal weight; grades 2 and 3 are regarded as obese – more than 20 per cent above the ideal weight.

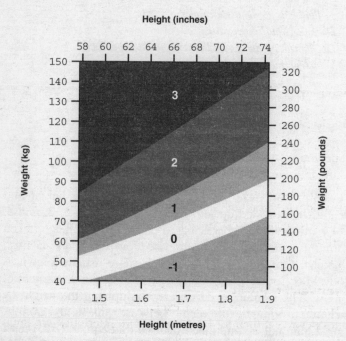

Height/weight chart showing the Quetelet grades of obesity

Results
Very overweight and unfit
If you are very overweight and you get puffed out easily, do little or no exercise and consider yourself unfit, you should begin by following the recommendations gradually, after checking with your doctor. Begin by exercising gently for 5–10 minutes per day, and build up gradually over a period of a month. Walking and swimming are good stamina-building exercises.

Moderately overweight and not as fit as you should be
If you are moderately overweight and similarly you get puffed easily, do little or no exercise and consider yourself unfit, you too should begin by exercising gently. If you are reasonably fit to begin with you will be able to increase your pace that much faster. Begin by going for a walk each day for half an hour or so. Gradually increase your pace to the point where you are walking briskly and you can feel your heart pumping away efficiently, but not to the point where you feel at all overwhelmed. A good way to tell whether or not you are overdoing it is that you should still be able to talk while you are exercising.

Mildly overweight and exercise occasionally
If you are a little overweight for your height and are doing some moderate exercise each week, but agree that it's not really optimum and you could be doing a lot better, you need to follow an 'improver' programme. This will involve stepping up your pace gradually and increasing the number of times you exercise per week. Swimming or aqua-fit are two good methods of exercise that get all your muscles working without experiencing the after-aches.

Overweight but fit
If you are overweight but are exercising happily at least four times per week, then far be it from me to interfere – continue with your routine while you follow the diet.

Enjoy your exercise time

The secret to sustaining your exercise programme is to select the kind of exercise you enjoy. If enjoyment is not the term you have ever used to describe the time you spend exercising, you will need to get yourself into the right frame of mind. Unless you come to enjoy the exercise regime you select, there isn't much hope of you sticking to it, is there? Some of us are sporty and others just aren't. There is little point arranging to play squash if you really dislike the game, or vowing to go for a jog each day if you hate running, so do select the type of exercise that you could grow to like.

There are a wide variety of exercises to choose from, but remember the aim of the activity is to get to the point of breathlessness. It is probably best to vary the type of exercise you do on different days of the week to prevent boredom. If you have a busy lifestyle it may not be possible for you to get to a specific exercise class each week. If budget is a factor then you should look at outdoor activities like walking, jogging and cycling. On bad weather days I find an exercise video an excellent way to begin my day, just stretching and dancing to my favourite music.

If you are not exercising in a class when you begin your chosen exercise routine:
- warm up slowly for the first few minutes
- continue until you reach the point of breathlessness
- this is the signal to begin the cool down process
- cool down gradually over a period of a few minutes, rather than stopping vigorous exercise suddenly.

Try to fit some exercise into your routine on a daily basis. You will need to chart the amount of exercise you do each day, on the daily charts provided in the Discovery Diet chapter. If you are nervous about sticking to an exercise routine, it may be best to plan out your week's activity in advance in your diary, or on a wall chart, and where possible arrange to exercise with a friend. Keep the benefits of exercise uppermost in your mind until your regime is firmly established. When you have reached the goal of doing four or five good sessions of exercise per week, work to maintain it, but don't exceed it on a regular basis. Believe it or not, too much exercise can be a strain on your joints and bad for your bones. Ballet dancers and athletes for example have more than their fair share of the bone-thinning disease osteoporosis.

Enjoy your time exercising. Regard it as time invested in yourself and it will pay dividends in terms of providing additional energy, increasing your productivity, and most of all making you look and feel good.

PART TWO

Health and Beauty in the Making

CHAPTER 7

Beauty and the feast

The fact that our diet has an effect on our bodily functions seems a reasonable proposition. But it goes further than that, for our diet and lifestyle have a profound effect on our outward appearance. If the victims of problems like acne, cellulite, dandruff and eczema knew that there were possible dietary solutions many of them would be beating a path to our door. These and many other skin, hair and nail conditions are often the underlying cause of great social embarrassment and introversion.

Let's look at some of the common problems and their simple solutions:

Acne

Acne is perhaps the commonest skin complaint in that most of us have had some experience of it during adolescence. Three types of 'spots' make up acne: the redheads or papules, the yellowheads or pustules and the blackheads or comedones. These usually appear on a background of inflamed red skin and are usually found on the face, back or shoulders.

How does it come about?

These three types of spot are manifestations of the inflammation, infection and resolution that occur in acne. Initially there is an increased sensitivity to hormones in the skin. Testosterone, which is present in both men and women, stimulates the production of sebum or grease. The ducts that carry this grease to the surface become blocked, get inflamed, then infected, they spot then either discharge themselves or resolve, leaving a blackhead behind which is the thickened remains of the infected pus of the yellowhead.

What's on offer at the surgery?

- Local applications of antiseptic, especially benzoyl peroxide, help by inhibiting the growth of bacteria and reducing sebum production. A local application of retinoic acid helps to unblock plugged follicles and is used when blackheads dominate.
- An antibiotic skin application or antibiotics by mouth. There is a variety of preparations with a success rate of around 75 per cent. Sometimes the bacteria become resistant to one antibiotic and a change is needed.
- A hormone-based treatment, using either the oral contraceptive pill or a combination of oestrogen with a small dose of an anti-testosterone preparation, is useful for more resistant cases in women.
- A powerful drug derived from vitamin A, 13-cis-retinoic acid, is highly effective as it inhibits the excessive production of sebum. It is only used by hospital specialists for those who have failed to respond to other treatments. As its use is associated with foetal abnormalities, women taking it should use contraception.

Simple self-help

- **Keep your skin clean** Clean your skin thoroughly, especially after using make-up.
- **Sunbathe** This often helps, though it may increase the number of blackheads.

- **Squeeze the blackheads** This is worthwhile provided that they are not pushed inward into the deeper layers of the skin.
- **Change your diet** Despite popular belief, no diet is of proven value in acne! For some, avoiding chocolate seems to help. It is possible that a low-fat diet (weight reducing if necessary) with high intakes of fruit and vegetables and a reduced intake of wheat might help some sufferers. Try the Discovery Diet on page 172 to see whether your acne is diet related.
- **Nutritional supplements** The only supplement of proven benefit is zinc but it is not as effective as antibiotics. A dose of 30 mg per day is needed and preferably taken at night to avoid nausea. Higher doses should only be taken under supervision. The herb Blue Flag also helps to resolve acne spots.

Eczema

This is predominantly an inherited condition, also known as atopic eczema or atopic dermatitis. It often starts in childhood and is linked to asthma and rhinitis. Itchy skin is the most noticeable feature, with the skin being red, scaly and dry. The distribution varies. It may be widespread or confined to the bends of the elbows and knees; it may affect just the face and neck, or settle in one or two other areas of the body. People with eczema are more prone to asthma, rhinitis, allergic reactions to drugs and abdominal symptoms due to food allergy.

Eczema has become increasingly common with estimates showing a doubling or trebling in prevalence in the UK since the Second World War. Having one or both parents affected by eczema or other allergies is relevant and additionally eczema has become more common in children from African and Asian families. Events in the first years of life and possibly exposure to environmental chemicals seem to be at work in determining who gets it.

How does it come about?

Eczema results from the body's failure to control certain

aspects of the immune system. A variety of different white cells which make up much of the immune system are normally busy fighting infections. In people with eczema this has failed to occur and the white cells themselves, or the proteins called antibodies that they produce, are targeted at a variety of everyday agents with which we all have contact. In practice it is allergy to these substances, which include house dust mites, foods and bacteria, that can be considered to be the cause of eczema. Possible triggers include:

- **Foods** Cows' milk, cows' cheese, hens' eggs, wheat, corn, yeast (bakers' and brewers'), fruits and nuts are all commonly implicated.
- **Infective agents** Bacteria that are frequently present on the skin surface, viruses including *Herpes simplex* and fungi including *Candida albicans,* can all play a part in eczema. Relief of symptoms may follow measures to treat these infections or reduce the amount of bacteria on the skin surface.
- **House dust-mite** This is a common allergen, and seems to be important in some cases of eczema as well as asthma.
- **Pollens and animals** may aggravate eczema in the susceptible individual.

What's on offer at the surgery?

- Your doctor can help in the identification of possible allergens by performing allergy tests, either blood tests or skin prick tests, and in the treatment of the skin condition itself.
- Steroid creams and ointments will, if the dose is high enough, damp down the irritation and rash.
- Moisturising agents will help with the dryness. Several good moisturisers are available without prescription; two examples are E 45 and Unguentum Merck, and may be all that is needed for dry, affected hands.
- Treatment for any associated infection. This applies especially to bacterial infection on the skin. Creams that combine antibiotics and steroids, antibiotics by mouth, or

antiseptic washes to add to the bath can all be used. Occasionally treatment of thrush (infection with *Candida albicans*) may help eczema.

- Other medicines include powerful drugs to alter the immune system and allergic response. One medicine is worthy of special mention for those with known food allergies. Nalcrom (oral cromoglycate capsules) is a drug that when taken by mouth is not absorbed from the gut but blocks the development of immediate allergy reactions that take place in the gut wall.
- Evening primrose oil can be prescribed by doctors in the UK (as Epogam), and is useful for very dry, widespread eczema. It is best combined with a high polyunsaturated fatty acid diet – see the food list on page 172.

Simple self-help

- **Change your diet** Try the Discovery Diet on page 172.
- **Avoid irritants** Many agents will worsen the eczema even though they are not the cause. Wear rubber gloves, cotton lined if necessary, when in contact with water. Use non-biological washing powders and liquids. For clothes that you wear next to your skin choose those made from cotton or silk as they are often less irritating.
- **Take some nutritional supplements** Deficiencies of vitamin B, zinc and the essential fatty acids can all affect skin quality. You may need to take supplements for two or three months to see the full effect. They are often usefully combined with supplements of evening primrose oil.
- **Go on holiday and get some sunshine** This is known to help for a number of possible reasons: the rest and relaxation are good for the immune system; there is a change in diet; the sunshine helps to kill off some of the surface bacteria; the warmth and light stimulate the skin's metabolism.
- **Reduce your exposure to house dust mite** as this can make eczema worse.
- **Treat any associated premenstrual syndrome**

Some of the dietary and self-help measures for PMS can sometimes benefit any associated eczema.

Hair loss

There are different patterns of hair loss in women and men. In men there is often a receding hairline, which is caused by the action of the male hormone testosterone. Women may occasionally experience this pattern, but more usually have either generalised diffuse hair loss or alopecia areata.

Alopecia areata involves discrete patches of hair loss that are completely bald. It is common in young adults and often recovers spontaneously. Treatment sometimes involves injections of steroids and always patience. There seems to be little that the patient can do to speed up the natural turn of events. Diffuse hair loss is exactly what it says it is, with generalised thinning and loss of hair from the top of the head. Generalised, often mild, scalp hair loss can also accompany any disease of the scalp such as psoriasis and eczema.

Research has shown that a large proportion of women reporting hair loss had low ferritin levels, compared with the levels generally found in women without hair loss. The main reason for this difference is due to the loss of blood during menstruation, which is just enough to cause a gradual depletion of iron stores, particularly in women who suffer with heavy periods, or eat little or no red meat.

What's on offer at the surgery?

Your doctor can investigate the cause by checking for:
- an under-active thyroid gland or other hormonal disturbance
- a pregnancy
- a fever or any severe illness
- a side-effect of drugs
- iron deficiency, even a mild lack of iron, might even follow blood donation.

Simple self-help

- Follow the Healthy Eating Plan on page 158.
- Take a supplement of iron if you are anaemic or if the haemoglobin level is normal but at the lower end (11.0–12.5mg/dl). A small supplement such as one tablet of ferrous sulphate taken daily for six months (as the recovery is slow) is safe and should correct any mild deficiency.
- Vitamin C works synergistically with iron, enhancing its absorption. Take a supplement of at least 1000mg a day, and ensure that you drink a glass of orange juice when taking your iron supplement.
- Supplements of zinc and multivitamins might be helpful. Again they will need to be taken for several months.

Nail problems

A number of minor nail problems are worth mentioning. Sometimes they indicate a nutritional problem.

- Brittle nails can be due to iron deficiency.
- Spoon-shaped or upturned nails can be due to iron deficiency or to repeated trauma.
- White spots on the nails were thought to be due to zinc deficiency but this is probably only occasionally the case. Repetitive minor trauma such as housework or use of a keyboard are more likely.
- Ridging of the nails can be due to eczema, psoriasis or other skin problems. Mild forms are quite common in normal individuals and have no nutritional significance.
- Fungal infections of the nails are common and respond well to the use of modern anti-fungal agents given either as local applications in the form of paint or as tablets. Additionally a supplement of zinc taken for three to six months might be helpful.

Eat yourself beautiful

Dry skin is perhaps caused by too much sun and wind without using creams or by eating an inadequate quantity of essential fatty acids. Vitamin A, necessary for cell membrane health, and vitamin E, which protects the skin cells from free radical damage, may be deficient. Eat green leafy vegetables, nuts and seeds and oily fish to help encourage healthy cells and give natural 'lubrication'. Apply vitamin E oil topically. Dry skin can be the result of insufficient fluids intake, so ensure at least six glasses of water are consumed per day.

Pimply skin on upper arms and thighs is often worse during the winter months when arms and thighs are not exposed to sunlight. They are often worsened by a deficiency of essential fatty acids and vitamin E, which are necessary for soft, smooth skin. Ensure an adequate intake of unsalted nuts and seeds, which provide good levels of vitamin E, and oily fish, which are rich in essential fatty acids.

Pale complexion This is not always a sign that you are unhealthy, as some people have a perfect but 'English Rose' complexion. However, a pale complexion can be due to anaemia, which is commonly experienced by menstruating women. Vegetarians are also susceptible, as they may be eating an inadequate diet, or one that is particularly low in iron and B12. These nutrients are most abundant in meat products and dairy foods, so it is easy for vegetarians to become deficient. Eat plenty of green leafy vegetables and nuts and seeds which are a good source of iron. Many cereals are fortified with iron and folic acid. Lean meat, eggs and to a lesser extent fish are good sources of B12. Vegetarians should concentrate on using fortified soya milk and consider taking a B complex vitamin supplement.

Psoriasis is a skin disorder characterised by rapid growth of cells, which take eight days to grow and mature, compared with a normal 28 days. Skin cells accumulate, creating a thick layer of dry flaky cells. It can manifest all over the body, particularly on the face and scalp. Nutritional therapy involves slowing down the cycle of cell growth and maturation, dependent on vitamin A, found in oily fish and low fat dairy products. Most cereals and breads are fortified with folic acid, and green vegetables are inherently rich in this vitamin. The minerals zinc and selenium are found in abundance in seafood and nuts and seeds, and calcium is found in low-fat dairy products, green leafy vegetables and nuts and seeds. The essential fatty acids help soften the skin cells, and make the cell membranes more flexible. Eat plenty of oily fish and nuts and seeds to ensure an adequate intake.

Rough pimply skin Drink plenty of water, at least six glasses each day, and ensure adequate intake of essential fats and the mineral zinc to improve skin health and reduce the dryness. Body brushing also helps, and apply good quality moisturising cream, preferably containing natural ingredients.

Cracking and peeling lips Concentrate on eating low-fat dairy products, lean meat, whole grains and green vegetables. Use a good quality lip balm, and concentrate on eating essential fatty acids to soften the skin.

Cracking at the corners of the mouth or corners of the eyes are associated with poor dietary intake of iron and vitamins B2 and B6. Vegetarians and women with heavy periods are susceptible to this condition, which can be resolved by eating iron from meat and non-meat sources. The B vitamins predominate in wholegrains, eggs, meat and dairy products. A good quality multivitamin and mineral supplement containing iron and B vitamins could be recommended.

Red greasy skin can be hormone related, which worsens premenstrually, and can be helped by taking a good multi-vitamin and mineral supplement like Optivite (available through WNAS mail order service, see page 317) which contains good levels of the B vitamins and zinc, necessary for skin health. Avoidance of saturated fats in the form of red meat and full-fat dairy products is suggested, together with keeping refined carbohydrates, like sugar and white bread and flour, to a minimum. Have plenty of fresh fruit and vegetables every day and drink at least six glasses of water.

Brittle nails, flattened upturned nails These are caused by iron deficiency due to heavy menstrual bleeding, an inadequate vegetarian diet or malabsorption of iron. Ensure you are eating plenty of fresh green leafy vegetables, nuts and seeds, and lean meat occasionally if not vegetarian.

A 'spare tyre' and fat stomach are often due to a genetic predisposition to storing fat around the stomach, which can make weight loss difficult. A lack of abdominal exercise can weaken muscle tone. Low oestrogen levels may be associated with this problem. Top up on phytoestrogens, oestrogens that occur mainly in plant food, including soya products, pulses and linseeds.

Cellulite Digestive problems, such as constipation, where toxins accumulate instead of being efficiently excreted, can increase cellulite levels. Increased levels of the female hormone oestrogen can worsen cellulite, which is often the reason why women experience heavier legs premenstrually. Caffeine can also worsen cellulite. Substitute normal tea with herbal teas like redbush or Rooibos tea and cereal-based coffee alternatives.

Saggy breasts Regular exercise for the pectoral muscles helps maintain firm breasts. Putting on weight often increases breast size, which means they are less likely to stay pert.

Stretch marks are often experienced during and after pregnancy, where the skin has stretched to accommodate the growing foetus. Zinc deficiency has been linked with stretch marks. Zinc is essential for the metabolism of vitamin A, which is necessary for the integrity of our skin cell membranes. Vitamin E taken in supplement form and applied topically can minimise the appearance of stretch marks. Zinc predominates in seafood and seeds, particularly pumpkin seeds. Eat plenty of whole grains and nuts and seeds to ensure an adequate vitamin E intake.

Thread veins and varicose veins are often hereditary. Thread veins are less of a problem, and don't really present with any pain or discomfort. Varicose veins can be worsened by long-term constipation where constant straining and pressure is placed on the bowel. Vitamin C and bioflavonoids, particularly rutin, are useful because of their ability to strengthen capillaries. Eat fresh fruit and vegetables and nibble orange peel which is a good source of bioflavonoids.

Wrinkles are caused by excess sunlight, particularly if you do not use protection in the form of a sunscreen and sunglasses. Eat plenty of fresh fruit and vegetables, particularly those that are dark green, red and yellow, which contain plenty of antioxidants. May also be due to a lack of selenium and zinc which are found in seafood and nuts and seeds.

Dandruff is thought to be caused by a fungal infection. It can be more prevalent in people with skin conditions like eczema and psoriasis. Eat plenty of essential fatty acids, found in oily fish, nuts and seeds. Biotin-rich foods, which include lean meat, dairy products and whole grains will help. Use anti-dandruff shampoos and perhaps apply evening primrose oil topically. Using tea tree shampoo, which has natural anti-fungal/bacterial properties, can also help.

Sore, smooth tongue, or recurrent mouth ulcers Consider food sensitivity, particularly where mouth ulcers are concerned. Try avoiding wheat and gluten in the form of bread, pasta, cakes and biscuits for six weeks – follow the Discovery Diet on page 172. A coated, sore tongue may also point to a food intolerance, worsened by sugary foods and refined carbohydrates.

Soft, bleeding, spongy gums Ensure good oral hygiene, brushing and flossing teeth twice daily to improve overall teeth and gum health. Eat plenty of vitamin C-rich fresh fruit and vegetables daily. Aim for at least four servings of vegetables, plus a salad and three pieces of fresh fruit. Visit your dentist if gum health doesn't improve. A supplement of CoQ10 helps oxygen distribution to the gums, as does brushing with fennel toothpaste.

Having this information certainly puts a different perspective on what passes our lips, for we can truly influence our appearance. Making changes still involves a good degree of willpower, followed by patience, as the resolution to the problems will not come about overnight. Realistically, it may take three or four months to see a big change, so you will need to persist. Keep a symptom diary, and grade the symptoms each day on a scale of 0 to 3, with 0 being equal to all clear, and 3 being equal to severe. In this way you can keep a track of your progress because, as time passes, it is sometimes hard to remember just how severe the problem once was.

CHAPTER 8

Period problems sorted

Our periods were not nicknamed 'the curse' for nothing. As our lives are longer and we have fewer children than previous generations, the majority of us have over 400 periods to cope with during our lifetime. What a nightmare! Those lucky individuals whose periods come and go unnoticed won't be phased by this, but in reality they are actually in the minority for at some stage in their lives most women suffer with either painful or heavy periods, which are often irregular. For some, periods can be so heavy and their timing so unpredictable that they wreck the social calendar for at least a week each month, and sometimes cause sufferers to be afraid to leave the house.

Conventional medical solutions have been offered to either mask or overcome period problems, all of which are either drug- or hormone-based. However, the medical profession has overlooked the weight of scientific evidence supporting the non-drug approach to overcoming period problems successfully. Tweaking your diet, taking scientifically-based nutritional and herbal supplements at the appropriate times and participating in a moderate exercise programme can make a huge difference to both the timing and flow of periods and can wipe out period pain altogether.

Case History

Sarena was a 26-year-old who had two children, the first one of which was born when she was 16 years old. She had been suffering with both constipation and heavy, painful periods and had been severely overweight since childhood.

'I must have tried every diet there is and had even resorted to taking slimming pills. Admittedly I lost weight, but then I put it all back on again. I got to the end of the line eventually when I couldn't even lose weight following the Weight Watchers diet strictly. I was 18 stone when I went to see Maryon, and only just over average height.

'I also suffered with constipation, which caused extreme and unbearable pain. I would be doubled over with cramps. My periods were really heavy and painful too, and I couldn't go to the loo at all before a period. It was a nightmare.

'I had PMS for years, migraine headaches and felt a compulsion to eat several bars of chocolate on the days before my period. I felt constantly tired and was always battling with throat infections.

'I consulted Maryon after reading one of her books. She gave me a programme to follow for a month. I had some difficulties at first as one of the supplements seemed to upset me, but once we had sorted this out there was no looking back.

'Within the first month I lost a stone. I couldn't believe it. The constipation and bloating went and the migraines were a lot better.

'By my second appointment I had lost another stone in weight. I was eating so much I couldn't believe the weight was just falling off me. My PMS was much easier and there was still no bloating or constipation.

'I continued with the recommendations and went on making progress. I even put my daughter on a wheat-free diet, as she was over-weight too. We both have so much more energy and feel so much better for it. I really thought I would be fat and constipated forever.'

Painful periods

Period pain usually affects younger women, but not exclusively, as periods can become painful later on in life. Period pain or to use the medical term, dysmenorrhoea, most often occurs because of excessive muscle contractions of the uterus with each period. Four common gynaecological problems may, however, cause the periods to become painful and they include:

- infection of the tubes or ovaries
- fibroids (an overgrowth of fibrous tissue)
- endometriosis, where the lining of the womb is found in other tissues such as the wall of the uterus or around the ovaries
- a deficiency of the mineral magnesium, the most commonly deficient nutrient in women of child-bearing age, which is needed for optimum muscle function.

While often no cause is found and the pain is attributable to the period, if you suffer with pain other than at period times, it is important to have a thorough check-up.

Period pain often lasts for the first 24 or 48 hours of the period and perhaps even for the day before the period begins. Period pain is often felt as mild to severe cramp-like pain or discomfort in the lower abdomen. It can also be felt as low back pain or aching down the legs and, when severe, can be accompanied by giddiness, faintness, nausea and even occasional vomiting. These other symptoms are probably due to the hormonal and chemical changes that occur with our periods.

Symptoms of premenstrual syndrome such as irritability, mood swings, depression or breast tenderness may also be present, but are not particularly related to the presence of period pains, although they may both have the same underlying nutritional cause.

What's on offer at the surgery?

A variety of treatments already exist that may be helpful, and could be suggested by your doctor when you seek advice.

- **Magnesium check** Have your red cell magnesium measured to see whether you have a deficiency. This is a simple blood test, and should be readily available.
- **Painkillers** Your doctor may recommend the use of certain types of painkillers or hormonal products. Some mild painkillers may not be very effective for severe pain but a more powerful kind, which are either prescribable (mefenamic acid-Ponstan) or are available on the advice of your pharmacist can be particularly useful. It may be necessary to try a number before finding the most effective one for you.
- **The oral contraceptive pill** A number of hormonal preparations are available but often the most useful, particularly in young women who require contraception, is the oral contraceptive pill. The more modern low-dose pills have much fewer side-effects than older preparations.
- **Iron** Your doctor can prescribe iron supplements if you are anaemic as well as suffering from painful periods.

Simple self-help

There are a number of avenues you can explore to help reduce painful periods:

- Physical exercise may sometimes be helpful with a variety of gynaecological problems, and may help your tolerance of pain. Try to exercise four or five times per week. During a painful period try to do some gentle yoga exercises instead of strenuous exercise.
- Heat seems to have a beneficial effect. Applying a hot water bottle or a thermal heat pad can be very soothing.
- Changing and improving your diet can help also with minor hormonal abnormalities, some of which are thought to underlie a variety of gynaecological problems. Ensure that you consume a well-balanced diet without an excessive amount of fatty foods, and with a good intake of fibre from

fruit and vegetables. This may help control hormone metabolism and can reduce some of the excessive hormonal swings that occur during the menstrual cycle. Try following the Healthy Eating Plan on page 158.

- Eat a diet rich in essential fatty acids, especially fish oils. Eat green leafy vegetables, unsalted nuts (except peanuts) and seeds, wholesome oils like sunflower, safflower, evening primrose and flax, and the oily fish including mackerel, herring, salmon, pilchards and sardines. Women with period pains are known to have a lower intake of these oils, which have anti-inflammatory and painkilling properties.

- Some minerals may also be helpful. Magnesium is particularly important in muscle and hormonal function. Its balance with calcium influences the contraction of uterine muscle and one study suggests that taking supplements may help reduce period pains. Good dietary sources of magnesium include all vegetables, especially the green leafy variety, nuts, seeds, beans, peas and lentils. (See page 300 for a fuller list of magnesium-rich foods). Sugar, sweets, cakes and biscuits are low in this important mineral. At the WNAS we recommend the use of supplements of magnesium amino acid chelate, which can be obtained through our mail order service. See page 317 for details.

Heavy periods

Heavy periods are very draining and can be a real social embarrassment. Believe it or not, the average blood loss for each menstrual period is only approximately 35ml, or just over 2 tablespoonsful. A heavy period, or menorrhaegia as it is technically known, constitutes a loss of 80ml (just over 5 tablespoonsful) of blood loss per period, which is considerably more than average. It is enormously difficult to assess the actual loss of blood during a period. Even studies that counted the number of sanitary towels or tampons that women use were inaccurate, as it was discovered that women change them after collecting differing amounts of blood.

Generally women find that their periods get heavier as they

grow older, particularly those who have had children. Apart from the sheer embarrassment and inconvenience of dealing with heavy periods, they can also suffer from iron deficiency anaemia.

Why do periods become heavy?

Excessive blood loss at period time is a problem for approximately 10 per cent of women of childbearing age, and there are many underlying causes.

- The presence of fibroids in the uterus can increase the flow of a period.
- A recently fitted IUD (contraceptive coil) can result in heavy periods, which usually settle down after the first few months.
- A hormonal imbalance in the body can result in heavy periods.
- An early miscarriage. Sometimes a woman may conceive without realising, but because it is an unviable pregnancy Mother Nature terminates it, in the form of what appears to be a very heavy period.
- And, according to my experience, heavy periods can often be caused by nutritional deficiencies.

What's on offer at the surgery?

If your periods become unmanageably heavy, or you have a sudden episode of flooding you should consult your doctor for advice. After taking a history of the problem, apart from prescribing drugs or hormones, your doctor should:

- Examine you to determine whether there are any fibroids present or any other physical abnormalities – in which case you would then be referred to a gynaecologist who would decide whether you needed minor surgery.
- Take some blood for a serum ferritin test to check whether your iron stores are in fact low, in which case you would need a course of iron.
- Remove your IUD, if you have one, to see whether that alters the flow.

Simple self-help

- Eat plenty of green leafy vegetables, liver, free-range eggs and other foods rich in iron.
- Take a good strong multivitamin and mineral supplement, like the scientifically-based supplement Optivite, with additional B vitamins and magnesium.
- Take at least 500mg of vitamin C with bioflavanoids together with an iron supplement to enhance absorption.
- Avoid too much wheat and bran, which contain phytic acid, a compound which inhibits iron absorption. Try following Phase One of the Discovery Diet – see page 178.

Irregular periods

Our periods were designed to be regular, somewhere between every 23 and 35 days. Each month the body should release eggs whose job it is to merge with a sperm . When this fails, a period arrives, approximately some two weeks later. After the first year, periods usually establish a pattern, which become the normal cycle, and for many this continues right up until their menopause. Others, particularly those who are underweight, athletes and dancers, experience irregular periods, or an absence of periods altogether, which means they are not releasing eggs. Over-exercising, excessive dieting, stress, or thyroid problems are all associated with the disappearance of a regular cycle, but equally, a hormonal imbalance with an underlying nutritional insufficiency may be the cause.

If you have had established periods but they have since disappeared there are a number of tests your doctor can perform, including thyroid and pituitary function, as these two glands are responsible for hormone function. Plus your doctor may also check your iron levels, and if there is any chance you may be pregnant, perform a pregnancy test.

Simple self-help

- Eat wholesome food at regular intervals throughout the day, and bear in mind that your calorie requirement is increased by up to 500 calories per day in the week before your period. Use the Healthy Eating Plan on page 158 as a guideline.

- As with heavy periods, take regular vitamin and mineral supplements.
- Introduce naturally occurring plant oestrogens, better known as phytoestrogens, to your diet. Phytoestrogen-rich foods are predominantly soya, linseeds and pulses. These compounds have a modulating effect on the body's own supply of oestrogen, which is useful for addressing this type of menstrual irregularity.
- Take a phytoestrogen-rich supplement like Novogen Redclover. This provides 40mg of isoflavones, which can be taken in conjunction with a phytoestrogen-rich diet to help balance hormone levels.
- Try the herbal supplement Agnus Castus, which has been used for centuries for its ability to regulate the menstrual cycle. The first major clinical study on its use was published in 1954, showing positive results on women with menstrual irregularities. It even helped missing periods to return. It is the fruit of the *Agnus castus* that contains essential oils, glycosides and flavonoids.
- Seek some help with sorting out any stressful situations that face you, or even counselling if you are bereaved or recently separated from your partner.
- If you are an athlete, a professional dancer or an exercise addict, work hard to ensure that you are meeting your calorie requirements.
- If your weight is low for your height and frame, actively work to increase your weight to the optimum range.
- A course of acupuncture may help to open the channels in the body and kick-start the menstrual cycle back into action.

In my years at the Women's Nutritional Advisory Service, I have noticed repeatedly that after following the WNAS programme periods arrive without pains or symptoms, and irregular periods tend to regulate. The good news is that in most cases it is perfectly possible to be in control of your periods rather than the other way around.

CHAPTER 9

An end to monthly misery

PMS

There can't be many medical conditions that are laughed about by men, but premenstrual syndrome (PMS) is certainly one of them. Amazingly, although women have suffered with PMS for centuries, not even twenty-first century doctors are able to agree on a cause, let alone a cure. Medical debate continues and current conventional medical treatments remain utterly inadequate.

PMS is often referred to as the Jekyll and Hyde Syndrome, for while some only suffer mild symptoms for a few days before the onset of their periods, PMS brings extraordinary suffering to millions of women and their families for approximately half of each menstruating year. A WNAS survey conducted in 1985 revealed that over 73 per cent of women of childbearing age in the UK admitted to suffering with PMS to some degree, with approximately seven million regularly suffering with severe to moderate symptoms. In the same year, from a survey of 1,000 sufferers, the WNAS discovered that 92 per cent felt that their relationships were affected adversely by their symptoms, 88 per cent felt violent and aggressive premenstrually, and a staggering 42 per cent of the sample contemplated suicide premenstrually, while 3 per cent actually attempted suicide.

A repeat survey conducted by the WNAS in 2001, revealed that the situation has become even worse. Ninety-seven per cent of sufferers now admit to experiencing mood swings, 92 per cent are craving sweet food, a staggering 99 per cent feel that PMS has affected their relationships and an additional 16 per cent of sufferers contemplate suicide premenstrually.

No emergency or other steps have been taken by the medical profession or the Department of Health to alleviate suffering following the launch of these devastating findings. On the contrary, on a Channel 4 documentary, not so long ago, two of the leading medical experts on PMS, Professor P.M.S. O'Brien, and Dr John Studd, went on record as saying that the solution to PMS was to take the 'happy' drug Prozac throughout the menstruating years, or to have a radical hysterectomy – which involves having your ovaries removed. It seems bizarre in the extreme to think that at a time when we can send women into space and clone new organs, the only offering that conventional medicine has for PMS would result in either a permanent state of zombyism or having a premature menopause, and the increased risks of osteoporosis and heart disease that accompany that scenario. What is also incredible is that these experts, as well as many others, have overlooked the fact that medical science also shows clearly that PMS can be overcome by non-drug means within a matter of months, without any side-effects.

Medical studies confirm, some of which have been conducted by the WNAS, that three key factors seem to contribute to PMS – the type of diet we consume, our level of exercise and our nutritional state.

Why do we get PMS?

A hormonal cycle requiring production of oestrogen and progesterone by the ovaries is necessary for the development of PMS. However, contrary to early theories, there is rarely a lack of either of these two hormones in the average PMS sufferer.

Research has shown us that over 50 per cent of women with PMS have low levels of magnesium, which is a mineral vital for normal brain chemical metabolism, hormone function and smooth-muscle control (the uterus and the gut are both smooth muscles). Other nutrients like B vitamins, zinc and essential fatty acids may also be in short supply.

Women often go through episodes in their lives that place extra nutritional demands on their bodies. Pregnancy and breastfeeding are two classic examples, where Mother Nature has deemed that the baby is served with nutrients first in order to develop and the mum is second in the queue. Therefore symptoms of PMS commonly get worse after pregnancy or weaning, or indeed may occur for the first time in a mother who is suffering from nutritional depletion.

Our bodies have very specific nutritional requirements. Just as our cars would not run well lacking oil or petrol, the brain will not be able to send out correct messages, and hormones will not be produced in adequate amounts at the appropriate time of the cycle when levels of important nutrients are at a low ebb.

The WNAS programme, which successfully helps the majority of women over their PMS, is designed to redress the balance, by putting back into the body what time and nature have taken out. In the short-term it will undoubtedly involve making certain dietary sacrifices until nutritional levels have been restored and symptoms overcome, but the general consensus is that the medium- to long-term plan is immensely enjoyable.

In addition to making dietary adjustments, the WNAS programme consists of taking regular exercise, and scientifically-based supplements (at least in the short-term) which act as a nutritional prop.

So many symptoms!

The symptoms of PMS are always cyclic, and there are some 150 variations. The most common 'mental' symptoms include anxiety, irritability, mood swings, nervous tension, depression, confusion, forgetfulness, crying and loss of sex drive. Some of the most common physical symptoms include breast tenderness, headaches, cravings for sweet food, abdominal bloating and fatigue.

Simple self-help

Try making the following changes to your diet, take some vitamin and mineral supplements and exercise regularly for the next three or four months, and see how you get on.

- Never miss a meal. You will need to eat little and often in order to maintain optimum blood sugar levels, and to keep a constant supply of good nutrients flowing through to the brain and the nervous system.

- In your premenstrual week, your calorie requirements increase by up to 500 additional calories per day. In order to avoid dips in blood sugar, and temptation to eat chocolate or other processed sweet food, you will need to eat both a wholesome mid-morning and a mid-afternoon snack as well as your breakfast, lunch and dinner (see page 162).

- Cut down on caffeine from ordinary tea, coffee, cola and chocolate, as the caffeine content can aggravate anxiety and irritability. Try one of the varieties of redbush tea or Rooibos, which is a natural tea substitute that looks just like tea when made with milk, as well as herbal teas and coffee substitutes. These are now available in many supermarkets as well as health food shops.

- Eat wholesome food little and often, especially during your premenstrual phase. Have wholesome snacks instead of chocolate including fresh or dried fruits, nuts, seeds, yoghurt, and oat or fruit snack bars.

- Eat an adequate amount of protein with your main meal each day, including lean meat, fish, chicken, eggs and a variety of vegetarian protein. Do not rely on excessive consumption of bread and pasta.

- Instead of table salt, which can cause bloating, use a potassium-rich salt substitute like LoSalt.

- Consume a daily salad with three portions of fruit and vegetables each day, particularly including green leafy vegetables.

- Take the daily supplement Optivite, which has been shown in clinical trials to normalise brain chemistry and hormone function.
- The herbs valerian and passiflora help to sooth anxiety and tension.
- Do at least three or four sessions of exercise each week, to the point of breathlessness, ensuring that you choose the sort of exercise that you enjoy.

There really is no need to go on suffering with PMS. At the WNAS we routinely help women to overcome their symptoms within the space of a few short months. You can read more about overcoming PMS in my book *No More PMS*, for details see page 335.

Case History

Harriet was a 22-year-old marketing assistant who had been suffering with constipation and PMS for four and eight years respectively.

'I felt like I had been suffering with PMS forever. I was emotional and tearful for what seemed like half of my life. I was aware that depression coloured my view of life, and each month I would experience suicidal thoughts. In desperation I accepted a hormone injection, but I lived to regret it as the mood swings got worse, my periods stopped and I put on masses of weight. I could almost go on listing my symptoms all day. I had acne before my period. I always felt very anxious and had little energy. My sex drive nose-dived and I had constant colds, infections and mouth ulcers. Apart from all that I felt fine!

'Amazingly, an aura reader at a festival gave me Maryon's contact details. I went along to her clinic because I was so desperate, but I didn't have particularly high hopes as I knew very little about her work.

'Within two weeks my constipation and pain were gone – I could hardly believe it – in fact I even got diarrhoea for a while until it settled down. I couldn't believe how much better I felt. It made a serious difference to the quality of my life. I had so much more energy even at that early stage.

'The anxiety and depression have cleared up. My food cravings disappeared and I lost weight. The degree of improvement in all my symptoms is nothing short of spectacular. I still find it hard to believe that getting better was so simple and I am so glad that I went to the festival that day, otherwise I might still be suffering.'

CHAPTER 10

Avoid headaches

Headaches can really spoil your fun. They often come on suddenly, choosing a time when you were hoping to feel at your best. The description most often used to illustrate the headaches is, 'It feels like a tight band around my head, like a skull cap' or 'as if a clamp or vice was squeezing my head'. Others feel as if their head is about to 'burst or explode', and they stress that there is a feeling of pressure as well as pain.

Tension headaches must be the most common human complaint. At least 80 per cent of the population suffer at some point, and they are essentially due to contractions of the muscles of the scalp, neck and face. It is primarily an adult problem, with women affected three times as often as men. Tension headache can vary from mild to severely disabling and can occur daily. It usually gets worse as the day goes by, but unlike migraine, is not associated with visual disturbance.

Tension headaches often come on when we are feeling stressed out, anxious or depressed. They are frequently associated with spasm of the muscles of the scalp, neck or shoulders. The cause is usually a combination of overwork, stress, lack of exercise or an emotional crisis of some sort, which causes the muscles to go into spasm.

Headaches often occur in the premenstrual week or on the day a period arrives. The oral contraceptive pill can also trigger headaches in some people.

Allowing yourself to get hungry can bring on a headache, just as going without the usual cups of tea and coffee can bring on a withdrawal headache.

When headaches are persistent it is important to ask your doctor to examine you physically, and to take a history of the problem. It is important to eliminate the possibility of the symptoms being anything other than a tension headache, and to determine whether the headache is caused by neck problems that might benefit from treatment by a cranial osteopath. It is important to have an examination and put your mind at rest, for anxiety about whether you may have an underlying brain haemorrhage will only serve to make the headaches worse!

Your doctor may suggest you take pain-killers, and while these may be helpful in the short-term, it is not ideal to go on taking them as they will only mask the symptoms. Long-term reliance on pain-killers can switch off the brain's natural ability to fight the headache. It is far better to explore and experiment with natural alternatives with a view to addressing the root cause of the headaches.

Simple self-help

- Eat a good diet. If your headaches are infrequent and mild to moderate you should follow the recommendations for the Healthy Eating Plan on page 158. The more severe and persistent headaches would respond better to the Discovery Diet on page 172, which you can phase in over the next few days.
- Avoid excessive amounts of tea, coffee and alcohol, and use the alternatives suggested on page 30.
- Identify any food allergies or sensitivities. Dairy products and caffeine have been implicated in the onset of headaches. However, caution is needed when cutting these foods out of the diet, because withdrawal symptoms can

manifest which can actually worsen headaches and induce feelings of nausea. The best advice is gradually to cut out the offending foods over a period of weeks.

- Avoid tyramine containing foods, which include chocolate, bananas, cheese, citrus fruit, peanut butter, pork, smoked fish, wine and yeast-containing products. Tyramine can cause blood pressure to rise, resulting in a dull headache.
- Never miss a meal, as low blood sugar can often precipitate a headache.
- Talk through any problems you face, and aim to get a workable solution underway.
- Learn to manage your time, so that you have time for regular relaxation (see page 148).
- Try to reorganise yourself so that you can avoid further stressful situations recurring (see page 111).
- Take regular exercise, preferably in the fresh air and sunlight when available (see page 52).
- Massage your own scalp, forehead, temples and ears regularly, or treat yourself to a regular massage. Use some of the gentler and more relaxing aromatherapy oils like lavender, melissa or geranium.
- Take daily supplements of strong multivitamins and minerals, with a strong B complex. Add an extra supplement of magnesium, in the region of 300mg per day, as magnesium acts as a muscle relaxant. It may take two or three months before it is fully effective.
- Try chewing some ginger, either root or crystallised, as this old remedy can often reverse the process of a headache if caught in time.
- The herb feverfew has been shown to be a helpful tool when attempting to overcome headaches. It is available from health food shops and through the WNAS mail order service detailed on page 317.
- When you feel the stress is getting the better of you, try going for a walk or doing some deep breathing.

CHAPTER 11

Curbing the food cravings

Who needs the excuse of Easter or Christmas when chocolate, crisps and sweets are available by the ton from supermarkets and garages 24 hours a day? Whether it is the smooth as silk 'mouth feel', the comfort it brings or its distinctive flavour, chocolate seems to be giving pleasure to ever increasing numbers of people in the UK. It is thought that one year's output of Cadbury's Creme Eggs weighs more that 1,500 African elephants. Nowadays a seriously alarming number of young people snack on chocolate and crisps instead of eating proper meals. So why is it that we are guzzling more junk food than ever before? Is it simply the skill of the ad man, or is there more to the story than meets the eye?

Comfort eating

Craving food, particularly chocolate, is very common, and affects approximately three-quarters of all women in the UK to some degree, with 60 per cent feeling that chocolate is a problem for them. Men succumb to cravings for chocolate too. It is not uncommon to hear of people who get into a routine of eating in excess of six bars of chocolate each day, sometimes whole packets of fun-size bars, or even a whole box of chocolates all in one sitting. While a little of what you fancy does you good, excessive consumption does little for our self-esteem, or our waistline.

Sugar craving questionnaire

The following questions relate to your consumption of sugar-containing foods over the last seven days. Before answering them, just spend a minute thinking back over the last week.

Now answer the questions. Total up your score then ring the grade that applies to you.

LOW none/1
MED 2 or 3
HIGH 4 or more

Over the last seven days:

How many chocolate bars or portions/servings of chocolate or sweets have you eaten?

1 ○   2 ○   3 ○

How many portions of cakes, desserts or puddings, or 'portions' of biscuits (1 biscuit counts as ¼ portion) have you eaten?

1 ○   2 ○   3 ○

How many cans or bottles of non-low-calorie soft drinks or servings of ice-cream have you eaten?

1 ○   2 ○   3 ○

How many portions have you eaten, either shop-bought or home-made, of foods containing sugar, e.g. fruit pies, desserts, custard?

1 ○   2 ○   3 ○

How many cups of tea, coffee, chocolate or other drinks *with sugar* did you consume per day?

1 ○   2 ○   3 ○

Low consumer 5   ○
Moderate consumer 6-10 ○
High consumer 11-15 ○

The craving mechanisms

The brain and nervous system require a constant supply of good nutrients in order to function normally. Eating nutritious food little and often will probably provide all that is needed, and indeed is the way we were designed to sustain ourselves. When we are busy and under pressure it is unlikely that we will shop for and prepare fresh food in the way that our grandmothers and aunts probably did. Clearly, many of us are not providing our bodies with the raw materials needed for normal function.

When we haven't eaten for a while or consumed much nutritious food our blood sugar levels drop. The brain, which requires glucose in order to function normally, sends out a red alert asking for more glucose, ideally in the form of nutritious food. Unfortunately, as we are not educated about nutrition, we often supply the body with refined sugar in the form of a sweet processed snack, or chocolate, which is largely composed of refined sugar, which doesn't contain any vitamins or minerals whatsoever, but does demand good nutrients in order to be metabolised. The result of eating the refined sugar snack is that the blood sugar levels shoot up rapidly, flooding the blood with sugar. The brain then sends another message to say that there is too much sugar in the blood, which triggers the release of the hormone insulin, whose function it is to drive the sugar back into the cells. It does this so efficiently that the blood sugar level then goes back to low again, and the whole cycle begins again as a result.

The trick is knowing how to break this cycle, which often develops into a real addiction, and just like alcohol, drugs or smoking, involves a period of withdrawal.

The secret ingredients

There are three specific nutrients which have been shown to be needed to maintain normal blood sugar control, but this has in fact remained a well-kept secret. They are:

- B vitamins (necessary for optimum function of the brain and the nervous system)
- Magnesium (which is also necessary for normal hormone function, and incidentally, is the most common nutritional deficiency amongst women of childbearing age)
- the trace element chromium (we are born with approximately $\frac{1}{16}$ of an ounce which lessens as the years go by).

Chromium, like magnesium and B vitamins, can be sourced in food, but we have to know where to look for them (see page 294). At the WNAS, where we have been treating chocoholics for over 17 years, we recommend a specially formulated nutritional supplement, which acts as a short-term nutritional prop to regulate blood sugar levels.

The preparation known as Normoglycaemia contains B vitamins, magnesium and chromium as well as a little vitamin C and is available through the WNAS mail order service which is detailed on page 317.

Helping yourself

The most recent report produced by The Committee on Dietary Reference Values recommends that we cut down our non-milk extrinsic sugars by 50 per cent – this includes any foods or drinks containing sugar. It is not necessarily an ideal recommendation, as it really depends on how much you were eating in the first place. However, it does present an achievable goal that should bring about substantial improvements in both dental and general health.

Dietary recommendations

- Consume nutritious food little and often to keep blood sugar levels constant. Eat breakfast, lunch and dinner each day, with a wholesome mid-morning and mid-afternoon snack to keep the blood sugar levels constant.
- Eat fresh home-cooked foods wherever possible.
- Eat foods that are intrinsically sweet like dried fruit, fresh fruit, nuts and seeds.
- Relax while you are eating and enjoy your food.
- Plan your meals and snacks in advance bearing in mind that calorie requirements are increased by up to 500 calories per day during the premenstrual week.
- Always shop for food *after* you have eaten.
- Cut down on tea and coffee. If these are consumed in large amounts they can also cause an increase in the release of insulin. Large amounts of sugar consumed in tea or coffee can contribute to an unstable blood glucose level. Try Rooibos or redbush tea, a herbal tea look-alike, and coffee substitutes that are available in health food shops.
- Concentrate on a diet rich in chromium, magnesium and vitamins B and C, including whole grains, chilli, black pepper, chicken, bell peppers.
- Reduce your intake of alcohol – apart from the fact that alcohol is high in calories, in excess it can cause liver damage, which can lead to significant hypoglycaemia (low blood sugar). Replacing a meal with two or three glasses of wine, for example, can cause a profound rise and subsequent fall in blood glucose levels, producing all the symptoms of hypoglycaemia.
- Take regular exercise. This is the one factor that can improve the control of blood sugar, as well as having many other health benefits. Exercise increases the sensitivity of the body's response to insulin, leading to smoother control of blood sugar levels. Ideally you should be doing at least four sessions of exercise per week to the point of breathlessness.

You will need to set aside some time for planning before you embark on the mission to reclaim your body and your brain. Make a menu plan for the week including snacks, and then go shopping, only buying what is on your list. If you haven't already got one, work out an exercise schedule, even if it is dancing or a workout video at home before the working day begins, and decide when you are going to steal the time for relaxation. It is wise to record how you feel about your physical and mental shape, and your chocolate habits, before you begin, so that when you go through the withdrawal symptoms in the first week you have a reminder to keep you on the straight and narrow. We have helped thousands of individuals successfully along this path over the years, so I can say from first-hand experience that there truly is a light at the end of the tunnel.

Case History

Jackie first came to see me in July 1999. She was suffering from terrible sugar cravings and had put on two stones in weight as a consequence of over-indulging. I remember her clearly because her dress buttoned at the back and was bulging at the seams. Not surprisingly she was feeling depressed, tense and fairly desperate. I put her on our programme, which included taking the supplement Normoglycaemia. By Christmas she was down to a size 12 from a 16, and her appearance has changed so much that her own brother didn't recognise her when he went to meet her at the station. She was a self-confessed chocoholic who no longer has any cravings at all. Plus she gave up caffeine and is able to sleep well at night. Her concentration has improved, her PMS has gone, her libido has returned and at her last appointment she took delight in telling me how great she now feels.

CHAPTER 12

Boost your natural energy

All too often we reach for stimulants to boost our energy levels and make us feel more 'alive'. This is a mistake because over-reliance on them can be addictive and destructive to our overall health.

Common stimulants typically used in the Western diet are caffeinated drinks, coffee, tea, cola and chocolate. Stimulants just give us a quick 'fix' of energy, in a similar way to sugar. Soon after the fix, energy levels drop and we reach for another coffee or bar of chocolate, and so the roller-coaster continues.

Fatigue

Many of us experience a drop in energy levels and episodes of fatigue for no apparent reason. In fact, the most common reason people visit their doctor is because they are feeling tired. While it is wise to check out chronic fatigue, unless there is a serious underlying cause to your lack of energy there is a great deal you can do to overcome the symptoms and restore your energy levels. A good diet, regular rest and relaxation, plus a daily multivitamin and mineral preparation with a few herbs thrown in will all help to boost your natural energy.

There are of course, different types of fatigue. Most of us

have, hopefully, experienced fatigue after a period of hard and fruitful work, and then noticed a return in our energy after a good night's sleep or a relaxing holiday. Some of us, however, suffer from fatigue day in, day out, despite the amount of sleep or rest we have. The causes of this problem vary from the physical to the psychological, and both aspects need to be considered in the majority of cases of significant fatigue.

It is estimated that up to 10 per cent of those with severe fatigue may actually have some underlying health problem. Some sufferers may have a physical illness which may not yet be fully developed, some may have recently experienced acute infection, and others may be mainly depressed. The first step must be to eliminate the possibility of any serious underlying cause *before* progressing to self-help measures.

How does it come about?

Causes of fatigue (not so serious)
- lack of sleep
- stress or overwork
- lack of physical fitness
- poor quality diet

Causes of fatigue (serious)
- physical illness, e.g. heart, liver or kidney disease
- after viral or other infection, e.g. glandular fever or 'flu
- depression
- rarely, a continuing infection like a tropical infection

Following illness

Fatigue can accompany or follow an illness such as a cold or 'flu or an infection. After the acute phase of the illness has passed fatigue may remain, and in some cases drags on for months and even years. This condition is sometimes called 'ME' or myalgic encephalomyelitis, which simply means inflammation of the muscles in the nervous tissue. It seems in some ways that the infection, after causing an acute illness, then goes into a slow or hidden phase, which can sometimes reappear. This is particularly true for the glandular fever virus, but may also be true of other viral infections. As well as fatigue, ME sufferers may also experience muscle aches and pains, giddiness, tingling in the nerves, especially of the hands and feet, headaches, and occasionally enlarged glands.

Other causes

Iron deficiency A large government-conducted survey published in 2000 showed that 26 per cent of all young women had low iron stores – a potential and important cause of fatigue. Iron deficiency is most likely in women who are having periods, particularly if they are heavy, and in vegetarians or people who don't consume much meat.

Vitamin B deficiency Mild deficiency of the B group of vitamins is also quite common, particularly in those who complain of anxiety, depression or mood changes. This may often accompany fatigue. Again, a poor diet, smoking, and drinking too much alcohol, are all significant risk factors for lack of vitamin B.

Magnesium deficiency The mineral magnesium has attracted considerable interest in recent years. This mineral is essential for nerve and muscle function. Intakes in the UK are acknowledged to be borderline or deficient in some 10 per cent or more of adults. The government survey of 2000 found low intakes of this mineral in 53 per cent of the sample. In our own surveys of women with PMS we have repeatedly found that over 50 per cent of women with PMS have low magnesium stores.

Good sources of magnesium are green leafy vegetables and most wholesome foods, while sugar, sweets and soft drinks contain virtually no magnesium.

Supplements of magnesium have been used successfully in the treatment of chronic fatigue syndrome, but it doesn't help everybody. Immune-boosting nutrients are important, including vitamin A, vitamin C, vitamin E, the herb echinacea and the trace element, zinc. Specialised fats and oils, as found in evening primrose oil and fish oil, have been used to help those with chronic fatigue.

Food intolerences and allergies In addition to deficiency of certain nutrients, sometimes other dietary problems can cause fatigue. There is evidence in those who have certain types of allergy, that fatigue may be one of the associated symptoms. Intolerance to certain foods seems to be a factor, and this can be suspected if there are symptoms of allergy, including eczema, asthma, nettle rash, migraine headaches and bowel problems. In one study, allergy to wheat protein was linked with increased complaints of fatigue, headaches and bowel problems. It is not known how commonly this is a cause of chronic fatigue, but it does seem to be worth considering.

Anxiety, depression and stress Symptoms such as anxiety and depression, often accompany fatigue. In fact many physical problems can also cause mental symptoms. Stress, in any form, may also aggravate mental symptoms, and even reduce the ability of the immune system to fight infection.

Overwork can result in appropriate tiredness and should not be confused with chronic fatigue. The solution must be to review your workload and find a way of making some changes. Working long hours and not eating wholesome food regularly is likely to make your blood glucose levels fall, which then makes you feel wiped out. The solution is to pay attention to your diet, get the balance right between work and play, and not to play so hard that it wears you out.

Being overweight can lower energy levels, leaving you feeling lethargic. Certain foods such as saturated (animal) fat and sugar can encourage weight gain as well as foods to which you may be intolerant. If you have been battling with your weight for some time, it is quite possible that your body is fighting against the food being eaten. When the digestive and immune systems are not functioning normally you are more likely to feel tired and run down.

Digestive disorders like irritable bowel syndrome can often result in reduced energy levels. Being constipated is a consequence of a sluggish bowel. When the bowels are not working efficiently, toxins build up within the body and can leave you feeling heavy, tired and generally out of sorts.

Following large meals Some people seem excessively tired and dopey just after a meal. Men seem particularly prone to this phenomenon, which is likely to be worse at lunch time or after a large meal and is aggravated by drinking alcohol. A smaller, lighter lunch, especially one of salad with meat, fish or vegetarian protein, avoiding alcohol and taking a 20 minute walk afterwards will usually prevent this form of transitory tiredness. The alternative is to have a siesta after your midday meal. It is not always practical, but this is what the Mediterraneans and the lions do, and is simply their response to the physiological need to rest while digesting a large meal.

Simple self-help

- To boost your energy levels follow the recommendations for the Healthy Eating Plan on page 158 and the suggested menu plans. If you suffer with persistent fatigue follow the Discovery Diet on page 172 for the next two months.
- Tidy up your diet by concentrating on good sources of magnesium – green leafy vegetables and most wholesome foods – and avoid sugar, sweets and soft drinks, which contain hardly any magnesium at all. Women with PMS often have low levels of magnesium, and it seems that the same is often true of people suffering from fatigue.
- Aim for three good meals, with nutritious between-meal snacks, such as fruit, nuts and raisins, a sandwich with cheese, meat or fish, or rye crackers and peanut butter, which give a more sustained rise in blood-sugar.

- Many other nutrients, if deficient, are known to affect the function of the immune system. These include vitamins A, C, E and the trace element, zinc. A healthy diet and a strong multivitamin supplement with 20 to 30mg of zinc should be adequate. Specialised fats and oils, as found in evening primrose oil and fish oil, have been used to help those with chronic fatigue. In one placebo-controlled trial a supplement of Efamarine at eight capsules daily helped a high proportion of those whose fatigue was post-infective in type. Again, this should be combined with eating healthily and possibly a multivitamin supplement.
- If you are feeling stressed it is important to find a workable way of overcoming the stressful factors and to spend a little time every day relaxing.
- Exercising regularly to the point of breathlessness and losing weight, if you are overweight, can also help mood and stimulate the immune system. Cardiovascular exercise, the type that gets your heart rate up, is excellent for boosting energy. The result is that your heart and blood vessels become more efficient, which improves their ability to carry oxygen to the cells as a wake-up call. You should only exercise regularly if your fatigue is mild and you have no underlying illness.
- Acupuncturists would regard symptoms of fatigue as a deficiency syndrome. The practitioner would be looking for deficiency of Qi or the life-force in the blood, and will treat the deficiency.

Fight fatigue
- Eat three meals a day, with wholesome snacks in between.
- Cut down on sugary foods, refined carbohydrates and chocolate.
- Eat three servings of fresh fruit per day.
- Eat three portions of fresh vegetables, including a green leafy vegetable, per day.
- Eat protein-rich foods at least once a day.

- Avoid bran and bran-based cereals and use corn and oat alternatives.
- Limit bread to 2–4 slices per day.
- Keep your alcohol intake down.
- Consume 300–600 ml of milk per day and 112–225g of cheese per week.
- Cut down on tea and coffee and try herbal teas and alternative coffees (see page 30).
- Enjoy your food.

CHAPTER 13

Control irritable bowel syndrome

What is IBS?

Irritable bowel syndrome is the modern name for a condition that was formerly known as spastic colon. It is the commonest gastric disorder, and accounts for almost 50 per cent of outpatients seen by British gastroenterologists each week.

IBS must be the commonest condition that is rarely discussed in public. Surveys on precisely how common it is vary between 10 and 25 per cent. Yet it is estimated that over 20 per cent of the UK population has been diagnosed with this problem, and probably at least as many again are suffering in silence, without consulting their doctor. Symptoms including abdominal bloating, wind, pain, constipation and or diarrhoea, can and do disrupt and spoil the quality of life and certainly inhibit the social lives of sufferers.

The occurrence of IBS occurs almost exclusively in civilised nations following a Western diet and lifestyle. A typical diet, consisting largely of refined and processed foods, over-consumption of one or two basic foods and hurried meals are just a few of the underlying causes. Researchers often refer to IBS as an acquired disease to which food and environmental factors are the most likely contributing factors, and if so, they are largely avoidable.

While the medical profession remains in deep dilemma over the diagnosis and treatment of IBS, to date they have very little to offer except drugs to mask the symptoms. The irony once again is that symptoms of IBS can be eradicated by making adjustments to our diet, lifestyle and improving nutrient levels in the body.

The symptoms of IBS

These include:

- constipation – opening the bowels infrequently, or hard stools
- diarrhoea – loose rather than just frequent stools
- alternating diarrhoea and constipation
- abdominal discomfort or pain
- abdominal bloating
- excessive wind
- mucus or slime in the stool
- nausea and loss of appetite
- indigestion

It is usual with IBS that patients will suffer with either diarrhoea or constipation, or a combination of the two, together with abdominal bloating and some discomfort or pain. These are the most common and typical symptoms.

How does it come about?

- **Age** Many people develop IBS symptoms in young to middle age, although approximately 12 per cent of those with IBS did experience symptoms during their childhood.
- **Operations** It has been observed that approximately 10 per cent of women are more likely to suffer symptoms of IBS following an operation on the abdomen as the reproductive organs are so closely positioned with the bowel. These operations can leave internal scar tissue, which is thought to be connected in some way to the onset of symptoms.
- **Radiotherapy** When the abdomen has been targeted by

radiotherapy, scarring can occur which may then once again produce symptoms of IBS.

- **Gastrointestinal infection** Most of us have experienced a severe tummy upset while on holiday or after eating a take-away meal. Sudden onset of diarrhoea, sometimes accompanied by pain and fever, can either be caused by bacteria or by a virus. Usually these upsets don't last for more than a few days, but sometimes the gut never seems to feel the same again, and symptoms of IBS develop.
- **Drugs** Some painkilling drugs can cause symptoms of IBS, either shortly after they are taken, or several months later. Antibiotics, certainly if taken in the long-term, can cause diarrhoea as a side-effect which may set up IBS-type symptoms in some. This seems to be due to a build up of *Candida albicans*, the organism responsible for thrush. This is often self-limiting and passes off, but for some it persists. Sometimes supplements of iron or multivitamins and minerals containing iron can irritate the gut also and produce symptoms of IBS.
- **Stress** There is now plenty of evidence to show that stress can worsen symptoms of IBS. The stress factors affect the muscles in the gut and can cause them to go into spasm, rendering the bowel inefficient, and causing pain. Chronic sufferers of IBS sometimes suffer with anxiety and depression, as their symptoms remain unresolved, which produces a vicious circle.
- **A change of diet** Food intolerances sometimes develop after a period of eating substantial quantities of the same food, or when new foods which are hard to digest are introduced.

What's on offer at the surgery?

IBS has become recognized as a condition in recent years and is often the diagnosis for young- to middle-aged patients, with abdominal pain or disturbance of bowel function. There are no tests to verify the diagnosis of IBS; it is often made on a balance of probabilities.

It is important to be screened by your doctor to eliminate the possibility of any sinister underlying cause to your symptoms.

Simple self-help

- Follow an exclusion diet, which is essentially avoidance of all commonly allergenic foods for a set period of time, which are then reintroduced one by one. The most frequently implicated foods are wheat, dairy, eggs and citrus foods. You can follow the Discovery Diet, which begins on page 172, in order to discover which foods aggravate your symptoms.

- Take a probiotic supplement which provides a standardised dose of the healthy bacteria *Lactobacillus acidophillus* and bifido bacteria. Eating live yoghurt might also be helpful, but supplements ensure a more precise dose. Most probiotics require refrigeration, but some are available on the market that do not have special storage requirements.

- If you are constipated add 1–2 tbsp of organic golden linseeds to your wheat-free breakfast cereal daily. They can be crushed and soaked in water or milk (soya or rice 'milk') for maximum efficiency. Crushing and soaking them reduces the risk of any discomfort associated such as bloating.

- Take supplements of magnesium amino acid chelate to improve bowel function if you suffer with constipation. Magnesium works by relaxing the smooth muscles of the gut. The WNAS recommends taking it 'to gut tolerance' which means that too much can result in loose stools. You can monitor and adjust your dose as you feel appropriate. Women often experience more constipation in the week leading up to their period.

- Aloe Vera is a good adjunct to following a specific dietary and supplement programme. Aloe Vera is used primarily to heal the digestive tract. Be aware of cheap inferior brands on the market, and choose one from a reputable manufacturer. Aloe Vera is available in liquid or gel form depending on the brand.

- Take some digestive enzymes. These function to mimic the natural enzymes secreted by the pancreas and stomach. Sometimes these are lacking in patients with IBS, especially those who suffer with chronic bloating and a feeling of fullness soon after eating even small quantities. These shouldn't be taken in the long-term as the body might lose its ability to produce these enzymes naturally.
- Charcoal tablets are quite a good standby for the immediate relief of bloating and discomfort. However do not take daily or at the same time as nutritional supplements because the charcoal can actually inhibit the absorption of nutrients.
- The herbal preparation of slippery elm has also been shown to soothe the gut, and the herb buchu helps to relieve wind and bloating.

The good news is that symptoms of IBS are both treatable and curable. We have great success in alleviating symptoms in our clinics. Constipation usually disappears within the first few weeks, along with the bloating and wind, and most cases of pain and diarrhoea are under control within a few months. So there genuinely is no need to continue to suffer. You can get further information about IBS from my book *No More IBS!* which is detailed on page 336.

Case History

Sarah was a 27-year-old administrator from Somerset, who was suffering with all sorts of problems including constipation, recurrent skin infections, depression, fatigue and premenstrual syndrome – interestingly she had a history of anaemia.

'I had been suffering from symptoms for years, in fact as a child I was hospitalised with pain from constipation. I had continuous bowel pain for as long as I could remember. I felt as if I had lost control of my body. If I wasn't craving cakes, sweets and chocolates, I was suffering with terrible acne. I regularly felt depressed anxious and weepy before my period, and too exhausted to make an effort to do anything but the essentials. My joints ached, I had swollen glands and generally felt a mess.

'I read Maryon's book on irritable bowel syndrome and decided to approach her for some help. Following my consultation I went on a pretty strict diet initially, because Maryon said I needed to give my body a rest. I ate mostly fruit, salad, vegetables and protein, with rice and corn products for carbohydrate, and I took the supplements that were prescribed.

'During the first month the constipation disappeared and amazingly, for the first time in my life, I was free of the bowel pain and the bloating. Even in the first cycle I had hardly any PMS and lots more energy. My skin had greatly improved, and my breast tenderness had almost gone too.

'As time went on I felt better and better. My IBS is totally under control. I never experience constipation any more. I no longer crave food or experience PMS. Even the scars on my face are clearing up and I have heaps of energy. I am so very grateful as I didn't think I would ever feel well again.'

CHAPTER 14

Curb the stress and beat the blues

S tress and depression are two of the most common conditions to affect millions of people at some time in their lives. Although there are sometimes underlying medical reasons for the symptoms, very often our diet and lifestyle play an enormous role, which is probably why stress and depression feature far more in our lives now than they did in times gone by.

So many of us live life in the fast lane but it inevitably has its drawbacks, and becoming stressed-out is one of them. Too much, or even insufficient, work, heaps of pressure at exam time, a relationship not running smoothly, or even a dispute can be the cause of us feeling stressed, depressed and wiped out. Some of us lose our appetite when we are under pressure, but many more turn to food for comfort. Unfortunately, it is often chocolate and other sweet food that we indulge in at this time in a subconscious effort to mimic the reward system that many of us had as children.

At times of stress we are so busy trying to keep up with our own shadow that any established exercise routine is likely to get put on the back burner. The increased calorie intake from junk food coupled with the reduced physical activity does little for us either mentally or physically. Our metabolic rate slows down and mentally we lose sight of the big picture. The net result is an undesirable merry-go-round with an expanding waistline coupled with low self-esteem, frustration, exasperation and then depression.

Breaking the cycle in order to salvage both your mind and body requires specific actions. First, addressing the source of the stress must be high on the priority list. Understanding the mechanisms of food cravings and dealing with them comes a close second (see Chapter 11 Curbing the food cravings), and last, but not least, you need to re-establish a regular exercise routine to speed up your metabolism and give you the benefit of those wonderful brain chemicals called endorphins, which help us to feel energised and improve our mood and the ability to handle stress.

Seasonal Affective Disorder (SAD) is another form of major depression, where sufferers are profoundly affected by the lack of sunlight that occurs in autumn and winter. This triggers biochemical changes in the brain, directed by the brain chemicals melatonin and serotonin, and leads to depression.

Stress or distress?

Our modern-day lifestyle undoubtedly has many benefits, provided we adopt a balanced approach to work, rest and play. Dealing with challenges as they present themselves is good for our morale. To a point, stress can actually be healthy, in that it keeps us alert and ready to face the day ahead. However, there is a fine line between stress and distress. Professor Hans Selye, the founder of modern research into stress, described it as, 'the rate of wear and tear on the body'. He distinguished between good stress and bad stress. Good stress can be reasonably healthy as it stretches us to capacity and keeps us on our toes. However, when we reach the point of overload the stress has an adverse effect, leaving many of us feeling overwhelmed and under par.

People have different ways of dealing with stress, and while some take it in their stride, others use methods of coping which result in undesirable symptoms. Weight gain, as a result of comfort eating, or bingeing, is a classic side effect of 'too-much-on-my-plate-syndrome', but it is not the only undesirable phenomenon. The effects of being overwhelmed can also include depression, migraine headaches, panic attacks, fatigue, irritable bowel syndrome, a nervous rash or even recurrent thrush, none of which are desirable.

The first warning for some of us could be a bout of 'flu, or the onset of headaches, as the stresses of life place extra strain on our immune system, perhaps also affecting our digestion and energy levels. Were we to re-evaluate the situation at this point, find and implement a solution to the problem, while investing time in getting our body back into shape, we might well be able to circumvent the health crisis brewing. Invariably, though, we get up from our sick bed and go into the ring for the next round, as many of us feel that we have to soldier on, no matter what. There does not seem to be an obvious alternative. Women are particularly prone to this form of martyrdom. So we continue until our body says 'no more'. We all have both physical and mental limits, and the body can tolerate only so much abuse.

The herb St John's Wort, which is otherwise known as *hypericum perforatum*, has been successfully used to treat depression for over 2,000 years. In Germany St John's Wort is prescribed by at least half of the doctors dealing with depression, and a study in the UK in 1997 found St John's Wort at a dose of one 900mg capsule per day to be as effective as standard antidepressants.

Depression creeps in

Unlike hormonally-related depression, which may come and go with our monthly cycle, a true depressive disorder persists, and the symptoms are not linked to the menstrual cycle, or lack of it.

Symptoms of clinical depression include:
• mood swings

- restlessness
- aches and pains
- fatigue or lack of energy
- suicidal thoughts
- agoraphobia
- disturbed sleep
- insomnia
- loss of interest in sex
- constipation
- weight loss or weight gain
- amenorrhoea (a lack of periods)

If you think you may be suffering with clinical depression it would be wise to consult your doctor as well as following the advice contained in this chapter.

How it comes about

Nutrition can be a very important factor in depression. Virtually any nutrient deficiency can result in depression, but there are some particularly vital nutrients for healthy mental function. Food nourishes both the body and the brain. In fact, the brain has first call on the available supply of nutrients, therefore the first effects of nutritional deficiencies are often mental symptoms.

Amino acids are the building blocks of protein, and precursors, or raw materials, for neurotransmitters. Neurotransmitters are chemical-like substances necessary for conducting messages. There are three amino acids that are most directly related to mood and depression: phenylalanine, tyrosine and tryptophan.

Tryptophan helps to raise levels of a naturally occurring chemical in the brain called serotonin, which has been found to be abnormally low in depressed people. Vitamin B3 is a co-factor in the conversion of tryptophan to serotonin so a good dietary intake with the addition of a supplement is necessary in the treatment of depression. Some foods, such as milk and turkey, contain an abundant supply of tryptophan and can act as antidepressants.

There are also plenty of foods that should be avoided, such as 'simple', highly refined carbohydrates and sugar, which can affect mental symptoms by causing blood sugar abnormalities and triggering depressive disorders. Excessive alcohol consumption can also cause depression, as it substantially decreases the ability of the body to extract nutrients from the food we eat.

Simple self-help

There is a great deal that you can do to help yourself over feelings of stress and depression without having to experience side-effects from drug therapy. Here are some tips to help keep stress at bay and your mood buoyant:

- Make sure you have some sacred time for yourself.
- Tell your family how you feel and ask for their support.
- If your stress comes from work, discuss with colleagues how you can make changes, or if you are self-employed you will need to re-evaluate.
- Try to get away, even if it's only for a few days.
- Learn not to take on too much.
- Prioritise your responsibilities and see if you can off-load or delegate some of the less important tasks.
- Work out an exercise schedule, even if it is dancing to a workout video at home before the working day begins.
- Eat regular wholesome meals and have a supply of nutritious snacks.
- Find 15 or 20 minutes each day to relax formally while you visualise yourself feeling serene, calm, happy and slim.
- Ask your partner or close friend to give you a massage.
- Watch an entertaining film or read a good book.
- Make sure you find things to laugh about.
- And make a point of singing in the bath!

Dietary recommendations:
- Consume nutritious food little and often to keep blood sugar levels constant. Eat breakfast, lunch and dinner each day, with a wholesome mid-morning and mid-afternoon

snack to keep the blood sugar levels constant. Follow the Healthy Eating Plan which begins on page 158.

- Eat fresh home-cooked foods wherever possible.
- Eat foods that are intrinsically sweet like dried fruit, fresh fruit, nuts and seeds.
- Relax while you are eating and enjoy your food.
- Plan your meals and snacks in advance, bearing in mind that calorie requirements are increased by up to 500 calories per day during the premenstrual week.
- Always shop for food *after* you have eaten.
- Cut down on tea and coffee – if reasonable quantities of these are consumed, they can also cause an increase in the release of insulin. Large amounts of sugar consumed in tea or coffee can contribute to an unstable blood glucose level. Try Rooibos or redbush tea and coffee substitutes instead. They are available in health food shops.

It is wise to record how stressed and depressed you feel before you begin your new regime, so that when you go through the withdrawal symptoms caused by dietary changes in the first week, you remember why you decided to make the changes in the first place. I have helped thousands of women successfully along this path over the years, so I can say from first-hand experience that there truly is a light at the end of the tunnel.

Case History

Susie was a 24-year-old who worked as a primary school teacher. When she came to see me she was suffering with severe panic attacks that were disrupting her life, and depression.

'I got really depressed with waves of panic one weekend so that I couldn't go in to work. I tried, but the panics were so severe that I couldn't get past the door. I had just finished a period at the time, but I didn't connect it. The irony of it all was that I had just been given extra responsibility of setting up a music department in our school. In theory it should have been a challenge that I would be pleased to take on, but the thought of it just made me more anxious. My smoking habit had also got out of control, with me smoking 30 to 40 cigarettes each day.

'I had a stable boyfriend by this time and he was very understanding, but I felt guilty as I couldn't lead a normal life. When I wasn't actually having a panic attack, I was worrying about having one. I couldn't face my journey to work as that involved going on the tube, which would send me into another panic attack. I was so exhausted when I got home from work each night, I simply couldn't face cooking or eating.

'I had a termination when I was 20 and developed premenstrual syndrome after that. My doctor prescribed Celeste, an oral contraceptive pill, which I took for two-and-a-half years, but when I came off it my symptoms got a lot worse and I developed depression and thrush.

'After reading the book *No More PMS!* I decided to contact Maryon Stewart to get some help. I went to see her in her clinic in London and explained the position. She gave me a programme to follow which was pretty strict. I had to make lots of changes to my diet initially, take supplements of Optivite, a special multivitamin and mineral preparation, a fairly large dose of evening primrose oil and some St John's Wort, to help with the depression. In addition I was told to get back to exercising, which I hadn't been doing for some time.

'By my first follow-up appointment, which was a month later, I was feeling less anxious, and the crying and depression was much better too. I cut down my smoking a bit and cut out chocolate, cakes and sweets. By the next appointment I was able to hold an assembly for 400 children without panicking, which I felt was a real achievement.

'I was feeling so much better and my relationship with my boyfriend had blossomed. In fact he proposed, and we got engaged on New Year's Day. I intended to stay on only a moderate amount of alcohol, but what with the Millennium and my engagement, I succumbed. I drank at least 30 units of alcohol in just a few days. I felt pretty awful for the rest of the month – the thrush came back and so did my PMS.

'I got my act together again after that as it made me realise just how important my programme was. I lost a stone in weight without trying and got back to feeling good again. So many people have commented about how different I look, and I know how different I feel. I really look forward to work now and am busy planning my wedding, which I realise would never have happened if I hadn't been lucky enough to find help.'

CHAPTER 15

Thrashing thrush

Most people associate thrush with a cottage-cheese-like vaginal infection, that is both stubborn and irritating. In fact, thrush occurs in other areas of the body, in the mouth, on the skin and in the gut, in both men and women. Thrush is simply an infection, usually with the organism *Candida albicans* present, which is the same bug that plays a part in the development of nappy rash in babies.

It is a very common bug with which we all have some contact, and the majority of cases resolve spontaneously. Surveys reveal that about 20 per cent of the normal population carry candida in the digestive tract without it causing problems, although some people, for a variety of reasons, are prone to repeated attacks. Interestingly, about half of those who assume they have thrush are suffering from a different type of infection, so it is best to get it checked out by your doctor.

Candida albicans grows best in warm, dark conditions and in the presence of sugar. Under these circumstances it changes from small round dormant spores to branching spores, and then to a branching structure called a mycelium which has the ability to invade and irritate our tissues.

In women, vaginal thrush causes irritation and a thick,

white, sticky discharge, which is different from the normal vaginal moisture that naturally increases at mid-cycle. Severe infections in women can cause swelling of the genital tissues and a rash that can spread out into the groin.

Men may develop soreness or redness on the penis, sometimes with a sticky white discharge. However, many men and women may carry small amounts of candida in the vagina or on the penis without any ill effects. In fact, candida is often kept in check by the presence of healthy non-disease-causing bacteria in both the vagina and the bowel.

In the mouth thrush causes a white sticky deposit on the tongue and elsewhere, which become sore. A slightly furred tongue without soreness is unlikely to be due to candida.

The skin can be infected too and this is usually in warm moist areas such as the groin, armpits or under the breasts. A red sore rash with spreading little red spots or 'satellites' at the edge of the rash is the usual appearance.

Why thrush persists

Candida organisms on the skin or possibly from the bowel provide a source of re-infection. Sometimes this comes from the male partner, and intercourse or use of a tampon may be factors in causing a break in the delicate tissues lining the vagina and allowing infection to develop.

Wearing trousers, tights, and nylon underwear may all promote the conditions that encourage the growth of candida. Local irritation can be aggravated by the use of some chemicals found in many toiletries, bath products, soaps and shampoos, so it may be necessary to avoid these.

There is also evidence that reactions to foods or yeast in the diet may cause a vaginal discharge. This might cause symptoms similar to thrush without candida being present, or the reaction may encourage the growth of candida already present. So, for some, a change to a healthier diet that excludes some foods can help symptoms of thrush. Following the Discovery Diet on page 172 will help you to determine whether your diet is making symptoms worse.

Why some suffer more than others

Although we may all get thrush occasionally, there are a whole list of circumstances which increase the chances of recurring outbreaks. Having low iron stores, which is not uncommon in young women, is a predisposing factor. If you have heavy periods or feel inappropriately tired it will be worth you asking your doctor to check your serum ferritin levels, which is a test that measures the iron stores in your body.

Low iron stores can reduce resistance to infection and lead to cracking at the corners of the mouth, making it easy for the infection to get started. A lack of zinc, vitamin B and even vitamin A have all been documented as reducing resistance to infection and leading to thrush.

Hormonal changes also encourage thrush. So being pregnant or even using a high dose oral contraceptive pill can increase the likelihood of an outbreak.

Various drugs encourage the growth of thrush. Antibiotics tend to kill off the 'good' bacteria, making it easier for candida to obtain a foothold. Steroid drugs, whether taken as tablets or with an inhaler, can also encourage the growth of candida.

Other medical conditions, such as thyroid or other hormone problems, and low blood calcium, can all lead to episodes of thrush, and the increased levels of sugar in the bloodstream of diabetics make it easy for the thrush organism to grow.

How to treat and prevent thrush

Your doctor will be able, by taking a swab, to confirm that you have thrush. He or she will also be able to determine whether you have low iron stores that need correcting and check your blood to make sure you are not suffering with any underlying medical problems. Once thrush has been confirmed there are a number of anti-fungal treatments available in the form of creams, tablets and pessaries.

These days many treatments for thrush are available over the counter at your local chemist, so if you are certain you are suffering with thrush you can purchase some pessaries or cream that may well alleviate the problem. Your pharmacist will be happy to advise you. Bear in mind, however, that all these treatments have a small failure rate and that if one treatment is not successful then another probably will be. The success rate for most standard anti-fungal treatments is 90 per cent.

The thrush should clear within three or four days. If not, see your GP or attend a local STD (Sexually Transmitted Disease) clinic. Such clinics are particularly well-equipped to identify the type of infection and the best form of treatment. You do not need to be referred by your doctor but can simply drop in.

Simple self-help

- Your diet should be low in sugar or sucrose, which means not adding sugar to tea and coffee, avoiding sweets, cakes, biscuits, chocolates and non-low-calorie soft drinks.

- For some a diet low in foods that are rich in yeast can help. Yeasty foods include alcoholic beverages (except gin and vodka), vinegar, pickled foods, yeast extract such as Marmite and many stock cubes, most packaged savoury foods including convenience meals and soups, and bread and buns and anything made from bakers' or brewers' yeast. Occasionally it may be necessary for the diet to be even more restricted than this, but fruit restriction is rarely needed. Follow the Discovery Diet which begins on page 172.

- It is important to address digestive abnormalities when treating candida, and the first point of action is to improve digestive secretions. Hydrochloric acid (secreted by the parietal cells in the lining of the stomach), pancreatic enzymes (which ensure efficient digestion of proteins and carbohydrates) and bile (secreted by the gall bladder) all inhibit the overgrowth of candida and prevent its penetration into the lining of the small of intestine. Specific supplements of hydrochloric acid and digestive enzymes can be taken in conjunction with an anti-candida diet, but advice should be sought from a professional nutritionist.

- Supplements may also be necessary. Consider a yeast-free multivitamin if you have recurrent thrush. A supplement of zinc, 20mg per day, can help, as can a supplement of iron such as 200mg ferrous sulphate (iron) once or twice a day, especially if heavy periods or anaemia are, or have been, problems.

- Capsules containing preparations of the healthy bacteria *Lactobacillus acidophillus* and related species are available and might help clear thrush from the gut (but not the vagina). Eating live yoghurt might also be helpful, and applying plain live yoghurt to the vagina is possibly beneficial but would be no substitute for anti-fungal medication.

- Caprylic acid is a naturally occurring fatty acid which has been reported to be an effective anti-fungal compound in the treatment of candida.

- Berberine-containing plants, including golden seal have shown natural antibiotic activity against bacteria and fungi, including candida.

- Garlic has demonstrated significant antifungal activity.

- Boosting the immune system by taking zinc, vitamin C and the herb echinacea can help with candida.

- Grapefruit seed extract is another natural agent possessing antibiotic and anti-fungal properties. All of these are available through the WNAS mail order service detailed on page 317.

Personal hygiene

- Avoid wearing restrictive clothing such as trousers, tights and synthetic underwear. Choose natural fabrics such as cotton or silk.

- Shower rather than bathe, and do not use perfumed soaps and other toiletries that might come into contact with your tail end. If you do have a bath, do not wash your hair at the same time.

- Dry yourself thoroughly after a bath or swimming.
- Do wash and change your underwear every day.
- When washing your clothes and underwear it may be preferable to use a non-biological washing liquid just in case traces of soap remain and contribute to the irritation.
- Use sanitary pads rather than tampons.
- Always wipe yourself from the front to the back so as to reduce the chance of infection from the bowel. If you are very sensitive, white unbleached toilet tissue may be a good idea.

Case History

Juliette was a 26-year-old computer programmer who had incredible cravings for chocolate, cakes and sweets or bread for at least two weeks each month.

'I felt disoriented and out of control. It was as if I moved into a bubble for two weeks each month, and would be severely depressed and very anxious. My sex drive went completely during this time, and I was impossible to live with.

'I had terrible cravings for chocolate, cakes and biscuits, as well as bread and cheese. I had constant thrush and cystitis, and suffered with constipation for half the month and diarrhoea for the other half, with unbearable wind and bloating. I had also been taking antibiotics for four years because of acne on my face.

'I saw Maryon in her clinic after reading one of her books. She gave me a programme to follow, which included taking Normoglycaemia to help control the cravings. I stopped taking the antibiotics, as I felt I had taken them for too long.

'By July, which was two months later, I was feeling brilliant, and my partner couldn't believe the transformation. He came with me to my first appointment and then went on two weeks holiday. He said he had dreaded coming back, but when he saw me he was startled by the change. Instead of being impossible to live with, I was even laughing and joking premenstrually. The confusion had gone and I felt fantastic.

'I haven't had any more thrush or cystitis, except once when I had a bit too much alcohol. I lost 10 lbs in weight, my nails are growing beautifully, and my skin is better than it ever was on antibiotics.

'Both my partner and I are over the moon.'

Juliette and her partner stayed together, she remained well and they have since had a baby.

CHAPTER 16

Goodbye to cystitis

O ver 50 per cent of women get cystitis at some point in their lives, but some unlucky souls seem to suffer with repeated attacks. It is simply an inflammation of the bladder caused by a bacterial infection or a mechanical disturbance in the area.

Vigorous sexual intercourse can be a trigger, which is why it became known as 'the honeymoon syndrome', but there are a number of other causes.

In approximately 50 per cent of cases the organism *E. coli* is present, which sometimes travels from the anus area. The bacteria penetrate the urethra and work their way into the bladder. Diaphragm users are also more prone to cystitis because of *E.coli*. Another factor is tight clothing, which can put unacceptable pressure on the urethra. Vaginal deodorants and disinfectants can also bring on symptoms, and caffeine affects the muscles of the bladder, aggravating symptoms of urgency.

Your doctor can test your urine to determine which sort of bacteria are present and whether they are sensitive to any particular types of antibiotics. Two-thirds of female sufferers recover naturally without antibiotics, and even after treatment with antibiotics symptoms can return.

Simple self-help

- If you use a diaphragm, and your symptoms are recurrent, try switching to an alternative method of contraception for a while.
- Drink plenty of liquids, particularly water, throughout the day. Aim to have the equivalent of a glass of water every hour while the symptoms are acute to flush your system through.
- Avoid drinking caffeine, and use alternative drinks, as coffee can make the bladder irritation worse (see page 30).
- Drink a few glasses of cranberry juice. Cranberry juice contains a compound called hippuric acid which actually inhibits the bacteria responsible for cystitis from adhering to the lining of the bladder and urinary tract. Look out for natural cranberry juice without added sugar, or mix a cranberry powder with water, as sugar has a detrimental effect on the immune system.
- Add a small amount of bicarbonate of soda to the water you drink; this can help to ease the symptoms by making your urine more alkaline.
- Follow the Healthy Eating Plan outlined on page 158.
- Strengthen the immune system to help prevent recurrent bouts of cystitis by taking garlic capsules and 25mg of zinc daily. Garlic, as well as being an immune enhancer, is a natural antibiotic.
- After sex and after a bowel movement wash yourself carefully with warm, unperfumed soapy water, wiping yourself from front to back to wash the germs away.
- Do not use feminine-fresh sprays but instead choose unperfumed bath products, as allergies can develop which can further inflame the urethra.
- Organic tampons and sanitary towels are preferable to the usual type and are becoming widely available in health food shops and even supermarkets.
- If there is blood in the urine, consult a medical practitioner for further diagnosis.
- Homoeopathic remedies like cantharis, staphisagria or apis may well bring relief.

- Herbal remedies, particularly cornsilk and marshmallow are useful for treating the inflammation, taken in conjunction with an anti-bacterial herb such as uva-ursi or buchu. It is best to take the anti-inflammatory herbs first to soothe the urinary tract, followed by the anti-bacterial herb. Take in tea form for a more potent effect.
- And finally, aromatherapy juniper oil can be used as part of a lower abdominal massage.

CHAPTER 17

Good mouth-keeping

Most of you will agree that truly looking good includes looking good when you open your mouth. Despite this a staggering 90 per cent of adults in the UK have gum disease and many suffer with bad breath. Amazingly just under one-third of people over the age of 16 in the UK have no natural teeth remaining and the vast majority of us have had tooth decay!

I suppose because of my dental background one of the first things I notice on meeting people is their teeth, and I have come to realise that the appearance of the teeth reveal an enormous amount about an individual. It's all very well wearing cool clothes and having expensive haircuts, but the condition of your teeth says a great deal about you, how you really care for yourself and how much attention you put on creating lasting impressions.

The most common diseases in the world are those of the mouth, such as tooth decay and gum disease, and amazingly they are both preventable with a little knowledge. As we only have one adult set of teeth and gums to see us through, it is in our interests to keep them looking good, especially as we seem to be living longer. There are many easy ways to do this, but first let's take a look at what lies behind your lips.

The teeth

Each tooth in the mouth contains a crown, which is the part visible in the mouth, and the root, which is anchored in a socket in the jawbone and covered by the gums. Teeth are composed of a number of different layers, and each serve a function.

Enamel covers the crown of the tooth and is the hardest structure the body. It reaches to just below the edge of the gum, and joins the cementum, which is the thin layer of bone-like tissue covering the root of the tooth and which helps to secure the tooth in its socket. Dentine is the hard, bright yellow, primarily non-living tissue that forms the bulk of the tooth. It reaches from the crown down through the roots. Finally, the pulp is the living centre of the tooth, which contains the nerves and blood vessels, and is therefore the part of the tooth that registers pain or thermal changes. The supporting structures of the teeth are known as the periodontium, and the gums are known as the gingiva.

Saliva

This is the watery fluid that is produced by salivary glands within the mouth. It is Mother Nature's own mouthwash. There are three pairs of glands in the mouth from which saliva is secreted. Among its other functions, saliva dilutes the amount of sugar-produced acid present in the mouth because of the calcium and phosphates it contains. Both these minerals in the saliva act to repair some of the damage done by dental decay.

Plaque

We all have a thin, sticky film, composed mainly of bacteria, called plaque, covering our teeth. It continually forms in the mouth and sticks on rough surfaces on the teeth. It is most commonly found in the little crevices between our teeth, on the backs of our teeth, and at the gum margin, where gums and teeth meet. Plaque feeds on sugary deposits from our diet, and the by-products of this cause both tooth decay and gum disease.

Teeth and gum problems

Tooth decay

When plaque is exposed to sugar from the diet, the bacteria contained in it convert the sugar into acids, which attack enamel on the teeth. After repeated acid attacks a cavity forms, which becomes deeper as more acid is released from the plaque. The cavity eventually works its way through the enamel and the dentine and into the pulp chamber, which then becomes infected with bacteria. The pain of toothache is generated from the pulp, and if nothing is done the pulp dies, and the infection then infiltrates the root of the tooth forming an abscess in the bone surrounding it.

Gingivitis

Plaque accumulates around the margins of the gum and the teeth, and between the teeth in the crevices, and if left to stagnate, produces poisons which in turn cause inflammation of the gums known as gingivitis. The gums become red, swollen and shiny and have a tendency to bleed easily. If you notice blood after you brush your teeth, you should consult your dentist.

People experience gingivitis when they take insufficient care with their oral hygiene and this is how the disease process begins. An improved cleaning routine can reverse the disease process, until, with age, the gums recede and bone is lost. Neither of these tissues, gums or bone, can be replaced once lost, and so it is vital to remove the plaque thoroughly each day in order to prevent diseases of the mouth.

Periodontitis

When plaque is left to stagnate it gradually absorbs calcium salts from the saliva and hardens to become calculus, or tartar.

This sits around the gum margin and is a constant source of inflammation to the tissues. As the disease progresses the calculus works its way down between the gum and the tooth into a pocket, and this stage is known as periodontitis.

Acute ulcerative gingivitis

This is an infection of the gums which is possibly bacterial in origin, but it seems it can also be attributed to some underlying nutritional cause usually at a time of particular stress. It was given the name 'trench mouth' following widespread outbreaks amongst soldiers who were sharing utensils in the trenches during the First World War. However, it is acknowledged that many of these soldiers were also suffering from scurvy, the result of severe vitamin C deficiency.

The gums become infected, turn a greyish colour, the top surface often rubs away leaving sore, painful patches, and it feels like something is wedged between your teeth, particularly the back teeth. As the surface of the gums is attacked and the cells die, a tremendous odour is created. This condition needs to be treated urgently with Flagyll, a special form of antibiotic. You would be feeling unwell enough to seek dental or medical advice if you were suffering, and not able to enjoy a meal because of the pain and soreness.

Cold sores

Following an initial attack of herpes in the mouth, the individual is likely to develop cold sores on the lips or face, which are secondary outbreaks of herpes simplex. They can be precipitated by numerous external factors:

- excessive sunshine
- emotional stress
- fatigue
- inadequate diet
- periods of ill health.

Simple self-help

- Make sure you are well nourished – follow the Healthy

Eating Plan on page 158.
- Get adequate sleep.
- Don't spend long periods of time sunbathing.
- Protect your lips with petroleum jelly in the sunlight, or other herbal creams like VyBrit, a German product which has shown to restrict the growth of a cold sore if caught in time, and seems to be as effective as pharmaceutical preparations like Zovirax. VyBrit can be obtained from the WNAS Mail Order service (see page 317).
- Avoid oral sex completely while you are infected.
- Try supplements of lysine, which is an amino acid found in foods. It can replace the chemically-related amino acid arginine, needed by the virus to replicate itself.
- Follow a diet rich in lysine and low in arginine. This means avoiding nuts, chocolate, carob, oats, wholewheat, and soya beans. Instead eat more fish, chicken, meats, milk, cheese, mung and other beans (but not soya).

Acute thrush

The digestive tract is like a hosepipe that leads from your mouth to your tail end. If thrush is present in one part of the tube, it can travel to other areas. Thrush can be found in the mouth, appearing as soft white masses on the surface of the tissue, which when scraped off, leave a red or bleeding patch. Occasionally it is a feature of diabetes, or can occur in a patient whose salivary glands are malfunctioning. It can be treated with antibiotics and you would be advised to follow the instructions given Chapter 15 Thrashing Thrush.

Mouth ulcers

Approximately 10 per cent of the population experience apthous ulcers (mouth ulcers) at some time. They are little sores that have a yellowish white appearance, and can appear singly or in crops. They also vary in size, but as a general rule the larger they are, the more pain they seem to cause. Apart from getting ulcers after you have hit your gum with a toothbrush, there is no recorded pattern to their occurrence. We do know that many women seem to get them in their premenstrual phase and that outbreaks occur when stress is abundant.

When nutrient levels in the body are in short supply, brain chemistry is often disturbed and the immune system, which protects us against problems like mouth ulcers, may become far less efficient. When nutrient levels are improved the outbreaks of ulcers diminish.

Through my work over the years I have observed a relationship between food sensitivities and mouth ulcerations. I very often find that women sensitive to wheat get a recurrence of ulcers when they try to reintroduce it into their diet.

Mouthwashes containing chlorhexidine or zinc are available at chemists and your doctor can prescribe hydrocortisone pellets or cream, which can be placed over the ulcerated areas to reduce the inflammation.

Simple self-help
- Get your diet in order. If you have PMS as well, follow the recommendations on page 83. If you suspect you may have some food allergies, follow the Discovery Diet which begins on page 172. If neither of these apply, then follow the recommendations for the Healthy Eating Plan on page 158.
- Take multivitamin and mineral supplements, and perhaps extra zinc and vitamin C.
- If the ulcers continue for more than four weeks, ask your doctor to examine them.

The good oral hygiene plan

Keep your breath fresh by brushing your teeth and gums carefully, twice a day, for at least three minutes each time. If your gums are really inflamed and sore, you can start by using a soft-headed brush, aiming to change over to a medium-headed brush to maintain the health of the gums. Gums need to be massaged to create a hard skin layer on the surface, a bit like that on the palms of your hands. Massage in little circles at the place where the gum and teeth meet, the gingival margin. If you are not sure about brushing techniques, check with your dentist or hygienist.

- You also need to floss between your teeth each day, in front of the mirror to ensure you don't damage the gums. This disturbs the plaque and food debris, which build up between the teeth, and are out of the reach of your toothbrush.
- Glide floss, which is recommended by the British Dental Association, should be used daily in conjunction with tooth brushing by anyone who is keen to adopt a thorough, comfortable and effective oral hygiene routine.
- Use a mouthwash to loosen the plaque before cleaning your teeth.
- Rinse your mouth with water after meals, taking care to swish the water around your mouth to loosen any remaining particles of food.
- Eat raw vegetables and fruit regularly as snacks like these exercise your gums, and unlike sweet processed carbohydrates, don't feed the plaque in your mouth.
- Drink lots of fluid to keep the saliva in your mouth flowing freely.
- Have routine checks with your dentist and hygienist at least every six months.
- Stop smoking.
- Brush daily with fennel or aloe vera with added coenzyme Q-10 toothpaste.
- Follow the recommendation for the Healthy Eating Plan on page 158, or if you suspect you may be suffering food intolerances, follow the recommendations for the Discovery Diet on page 172.
- Take supplements of multivitamins and minerals and additional vitamin C, at least 1g per day.

Your smile says so much about you, so make sure you take proper care of your gums and your teeth in order to do yourself justice.

CHAPTER 18

Off the hook – addiction

My general philosophy in life is that 'a little of what you fancy does you good'. This seems to work well until we forget the importance of the word 'little'. When our intakes or use of the things that are not very good for our body increase because of stress, boredom or social pressure, we begin to run into trouble, which can affect how we feel and how we look. It's a pity that it is those things that we enjoy the most that often turn out to be bad for us. We simply were not designed to smoke tobacco and other substances or drink coffee, alcohol and cola until it comes out of our ears.

If you are in good health, moderation should be your rule. However, when you feel less than good, or are having a personal health crisis, it may be necessary to make some sacrifices. Often the thought of making the changes is worse than actually taking the plunge. Surprisingly, people find the alternatives relatively acceptable once they have taken the plunge. They soon decide they prefer the health benefits and quickly feel delighted to be free from the 'addiction' or dependency. These may sound strong words, but it is not uncommon to find that the withdrawal of regular, but relatively small, amounts of caffeine – one or two mugs per day, say – can result in withdrawal headaches and other symptoms.

Often the biggest hurdles to overcome are social, for smoking and drinking, be it alcohol, tea or coffee, are often part of our social agenda. In fact, they are often the linchpin for the occasion – friends may invite you out for a drink or over for a coffee, so concern about how they might react is perfectly valid. You may worry they'll make fun of you, or that you'll be the only one not enjoying yourself. In reality, most of us are in the same boat. Our bodies will only stand so much abuse. Bite the bullet and who knows, maybe once you have sorted yourself out you can pass the word on to others. They will undoubtedly respect you for it in the end.

Let us look at these social substances individually and see just where they fall down.

Caffeine

Many of us have become slowly dependent on caffeine over the years because that was the example set for us. Like other European countries we are evolving into a café society. We have more opportunities to consume caffeine, sometimes without even knowing it. You will find caffeine in coffee and tea as you might expect, but also in chocolate, chocolate drinks, cocoa, cola-based drinks, Lucozade, Lemsip, some painkillers, and the new generation of drinks like Red Bull, Red Kick and Virgin Energy.

Caffeine is one of the substances known as methylxanthines, which act as both physical and mental stimulants. Although small amounts of caffeine can be of benefit in waking us up and stimulating our thought processes, it can have many adverse effects when used to excess. We know that caffeine worsens nervous tension, anxiety, insomnia and aggravates breast tenderness. It can also make us feel restless, nervous, with a rapid pulse and palpitations. Over the years caffeine has also been linked to heart disease, high blood pressure and even infertility.

If you have been consuming a significant amount of caffeine, it is likely that you will probably experience withdrawal symptoms when trying to kick the habit, rather like the symptoms produced by alcohol or nicotine withdrawal. If you depend on the caffeine buzz, then the road to good health will undoubtedly involve reducing your intake.

Coffee

Coffee is the most widely used drug of our time. We are consuming more coffee than ever before. Since 1950 the consumption of coffee in the UK, for instance, has increased four-fold. There are many unacknowledged 'addicts' who would find it a challenge to give up, and even foregoing that last cup can produce symptoms of restlessness, nervous tension and headaches.

Ground coffee contains approximately 250mg of caffeine per mug, and a mug of instant coffee roughly 150mg. When we are well, moderate doses of up to 250mg may be acceptable, but large doses can produce symptoms that could be mistaken for anxiety neurosis, including headaches, tremors, nausea and diarrhoea.

Weaning yourself off coffee can sometimes be a traumatic experience, but sadly there is no real shortcut. Cutting down gradually over a few weeks is the best option, and even when parting with those last few cups, set aside a few days so that you can hide away if you get a bad headache or really, really uptight.

How to kick the habit

- Reduce your intake gradually over the space of a week or two.
- Limit yourself to no more than two cups of decaffeinated coffee per day.
- Try some of the alternative drinks like Barleycup, dandelion coffee, or No Caf, which you can obtain from health-food shops.
- If you enjoy filter coffee, you can still use your filter, but

with decaffeinated versions or with roasted dandelion root instead, which you can also buy from health-food shops. Simply grind it and put it through a filter, treating it just like ground coffee. It makes a 'coffee-like' strong malted drink.

Tea

The bad news is that tea, the great British beverage, is not much better for us than coffee. It contains about 70mg of caffeine per cup and approximately 100mg per mug. However, it also contains tannin, another nasty, which inhibits the absorption of nutrients, zinc and iron in particular. Excesses of tea can produce the same withdrawal symptoms as coffee, but tea also can cause constipation.

Drinking tea with a meal will reduce the absorption of iron from vegetarian sources by one-third, whereas a glass of fresh orange juice, rich in vitamin C, would increase the iron absorption two-fold. Vegetarians and vegans need their iron, so drinking anything other than small amounts of weak tea, in between meals, may mean they risk becoming iron deficient.

What's the alternative?

Herbal teas are a good substitute. Unlike conventional Indian or Chinese leaf tea, most of the herbal varieties are free of caffeine and tannin, and can be both cleansing and relaxing. A good herbal tea look-alike is Rooibos or redbush tea, which look just like ordinary tea when made with milk. As an added bonus it contains a muscle relaxant and has been used in trials on babies with colic. Many of my patients prefer it to ordinary tea after a few weeks, but it does take a while to get used to it. The good news is that it has recently become available in Sainsbury's and Waitrose and it probably won't be too long before the other supermarkets give it shelf space. Apart from this there are many delicious varieties of herbal tea, and these days you can buy single sachets to try, which means you don't get left with a box full of teabags you dislike. My current favourites, apart from Rooibos, which is also nice black with lemon or ginger, are lemon and ginger, mixed berry and fennel.

Caffeinated fizzy drinks

We used to have only cola-based drinks to contend with, but these days there are caffeinated drinks such as Red Bull and Virgin Energy. Apart from caffeine there is also sugar to consider, approximately eight teaspoons per can of cola, or the chemical substitutes, and other additives. Sadly many young people get hooked on these drinks early on in life.

We are all much better off with the healthy varieties of fizzy drink, which thankfully are given substantial space on our supermarket shelves. Appletise, Amé, and Irish Spring are all good examples. Or you can simply dilute some fruit juice with some fizzy bottled water yourself.

If you have been a large consumer of the caffeined varieties, you will have to follow the weaning instructions for coffee. We have had patients who consume two or more litres of cola per day, and know that the withdrawal symptoms are likely to be quite similar.

Decaffeinated drinks

Decaffeinated drinks usually still contain small amounts of caffeine as well as other members of the methylxanthine family, and decaffeinated tea also contains tannin. The regulations for decaffeinated cola are no more than 125mg per litre.

The decaffeination process uses one of two methods, either water and carbon dioxide, or the Swiss water process which uses hot water, charcoal and the use of chemical solvents. In the latter process small residues of chemicals remain, but they are minimal, so decaffeinated drinks are better but not marvellous. At the WNAS we recommend restricting decaffeinated drinks to no more than two mugs per day.

Alcohol

While small amounts of alcohol on a regular basis are not

harmful, unless we are planning a pregnancy, or are already pregnant, we know that alcohol knocks most nutrients sideways, and big consumers are putting themselves seriously at risk of all manner of medical problems.

The bad news is that, over the years, alcohol in excess destroys body tissue, and can cause or contribute to a long list of awful diseases, including:

- cardiovascular diseases
- digestive disorders
- inflammation and ulceration of the lining of the digestive tract
- liver disease
- cancer, including breast cancer
- brain degeneration
- miscarriages
- damage to unborn children
- heavy drinking can be a risk factor for the bone thinning disease, osteoporosis.

Amazingly, one-third of divorce petitions cite alcohol as a contributory factor. It is absolutely true that people under stress do sometimes hit the bottle in order to escape from reality, and as most of the above conditions come on gradually, we often don't perceive the real dangers of alcohol until it is too late. If your drinking has been escalating slowly it is advisable to seek help. It is important to keep our alcohol intake to around or less than the recommended limits which are no more than 14 units per week for the girls and 21 units per week for the boys. One unit is equivalent to either one average glass of wine, one measure of spirits or half a pint of either lager or beer.

Tobacco

Can you believe that earlier this century cigarettes were actually recommended by doctors as safe and therapeutic? More recent research, as most of us are only too aware, has shown that in all but a few circumstances, cigarettes are bad for our general health. Smoking during pregnancy can also harm the growing baby, as well as cause increased bone loss throughout our lifetime.

Despite government health warnings and health-promotion campaigns, the number of young people who still start to smoke is enormous. Although research shows that the better-educated women have cut back, more and more younger women, who are perhaps not so well educated, are still puffing away. Despite all the health warnings, it is still considered cool to smoke, and it feels so grown-up!

Kicking the habit

Giving up smoking has never been easy. The first step is to make the decision to quit, knowing that you may well experience true withdrawal symptoms, just as drug addicts and alcoholics do when they try to stop. Here is a plan to help you:

- Choose a day on which to give up, and write down the date.
- On the day before, smoke as many cigarettes as you can until you feel sick. Make sure you stub them out in the same dirty ashtray.
- Go to the library and get a book that contains pictures of the consequences of smoking.
- On the morning of your chosen day, pour yourself a glass of freshly squeezed orange juice, then sit and write down all the reasons for your decision to give up smoking.
- Pin your list of reasons up on the wall so that you can read it at weak moments.
- Put your cigarettes away in a drawer, and tell yourself you can have one whenever you like.
- When you crave a cigarette, tell yourself you can have one but first consider the reasons why you decided to quit. Make a new decision not to light up.
- Go shopping and stock up with some of your favourite wholesome food, including some fruit and some raw vegetables and dips.
- Tell your close friends and family that you are giving up smoking.

- Take a good multivitamin and mineral pill each day, in addition to improving your diet.
- Try to avoid situations that are likely to make you feel like lighting up. For example, drink fruit juice instead of alcohol.
- If possible, go away for a few days to help you break your daily routine.
- Chew some sugar-free gum rather than sweets or chocolate.
- Put the handle of your toothbrush in your mouth whenever you miss your hand-to-mouth habit.
- Each time you feel you need a cigarette, stop, relax and breathe deeply, so that you get a good supply of oxygen into your lungs.
- Join a gym, and make sure you exercise regularly.
- Don't spend evenings alone, instead arrange to go to the cinema, or out for a walk.
- If you feel edgy in the evenings, have a few early nights.
- Keep a progress chart, ticking each day that you have remained a non-smoker.
- Save your cigarette money in a jar, and spend it on treats for yourself.
- Practise some formal relaxation like yoga or meditation.
- If you have a partner, ask for a massage when you feel tense or a bit ratty.
- Picture your lungs recovering now that they are smoke-free.

It is never too late to give up smoking. Whenever you do decide to give up you will be helping to keep your skin in better shape, you won't smell of stale smoke, and, once you are through the withdrawal phase, you will feel so much better in yourself. If you find it difficult to quit, contact one of the organisations listed in Useful addresses on page 322 and read some of the suggested books on page 335.

Street drugs

These have become increasingly popular in the last 15 or 20

years. They are readily available and can sometimes be a tempting option for those whose lives are either not going so well or are not considered to be very exciting. Women of child-bearing age should avoid all street drugs as they undoubtedly harm a growing baby, and in some case babies are born addicted. Drug users, even more so than smokers, tend to have a less nutritious diet than non-users, and are not so concerned about preserving their health, as they are in the process of spoiling it anyway.

Marijuana and cannabis are both widely used and are products of the hemp plant. The pro-marijuana lobby claims that it is as safe as smoking cigarettes or drinking alcohol. While marijuana does seem to have some medicinal uses, and it may well be legalised in the not too distant future, there are too many studies that show that regular use adversely affects our short-term memory as well as other aspects of our brain function.

When we run into health difficulties, be they physical or emotional, our body depends on us to clean up our act so that the immune system can function properly and do its job. The body has exceptional natural healing powers, but you wouldn't expect a wound to heal with a nail in it, any more than you can expect to be well without treating your body with respect.

It must be preferable to work on stimulating the brain chemicals that give us a high naturally. Being successful in life, eating exotic food and taking regular aerobic exercise can all help to give you that desirable feel-good factor. So think before you indulge, and give the natural route a try at least. If you feel you have become dependent on a particular drug or are getting into bad habits you can contact Drugaid for some confidential advice and guidance. See page 320 for details.

CHAPTER 19

Learn to love yourself

When it comes to self-image, the majority of us should be awarded a Masters Degree in fault picking. I have yet to meet anyone who can't find a multitude of things wrong with them, be it physical or otherwise. Their hair is the wrong shade, or it's curly instead of straight or vice versa. Maybe their nose is too long, the eyes too small or the wrong colour, and as for their figure or physique, well that's a disaster too because it's not the right shape. Maybe we feel that we are never as full of personality as others we know, nor as intelligent, and so it goes on.

How much do you like yourself?

The truth is that none of us is truly perfect, and most of us will probably never be entirely satisfied with our lot. However, while there is always room for improvement, we should not overlook the positive attributes that make us what we are. You have probably never stopped to make a list of the things you and others like about yourself. Well now is the time. Write down five things you like about your body and another five things you like about yourself.

Things I like about my body	Things I like about myself
1.	1. . . . .
2.	2. . . . .
3.	3. . . . .
4.	4. . . . .
5.	5. . . . .

Why is it that for every positive point we note about ourselves, we can think of at least two negative factors without much effort? I can't honestly answer that question except to guess that it seems to be part of the human condition. What I do appreciate, however, is the importance of liking yourself sufficiently to appear attractive to others, not just in a physical way. For there is no doubt that others are attracted to positive, outgoing, confident and successful individuals.

Be positive

Being outgoing and optimistic is far more likely to bring success than spending time on introspection. There is plenty of evidence to confirm that those who clearly believe they will be successful usually are. So if you are short on confidence make a point of indulging in some positive thinking for 10 minutes each morning, before your day begins, and again just before you drop off to sleep at night. Spend the time imagining good things happening to you. Maybe it's success with the opposite sex that you are seeking, or just good friendships. Perhaps your daydreams will centre around success in your studies or at work, or it may be that you want to look and feel attractive to others. Whatever you decide to focus on make the images in your mind so realistic that you can actually feel that you are the experiencing the situation. It may take a bit of practice, but once you get the hang of it, it is like watching a movie.

Pat yourself on the back

Another important daily practice is to keep a note of your achievements, no matter how small. It is far too easy to move on to the next thing, or even the next day, without acknowledging what you have actually accomplished. Once again, we are generally quick to fixate on the negative, our mistakes and things that perhaps we later regret. Making time to review your successes will pay dividends, as being satisfied with our performance makes us more confident and outgoing. Get yourself a notebook, which you can dedicate to this activity, and write in it on a daily basis as you would a diary.

Make yourself proud

Life can be so demanding that it's all too easy to go from day to day fulfilling your own needs without stopping to consider the needs of others. In my experience, a big part of liking yourself is the reward that comes from helping to make the lives of others more pleasant. Being a good friend, listening to others when they need to talk and being supportive are all tremendously valuable activities. Make a point of doing something nice for someone each day and make a note of it on your list of daily achievements. You will be surprised by the feedback you get from treating others as you would like to be treated yourself.

Make time for yourself

Making time for yourself is not just a nice idea, it is a necessity, especially if you lead and full and demanding life. Often, with the best will in the world, our new years' resolutions to exercise regularly and make more time for relaxation go out of the window at the first sign of a hiccup to our routine.

Stress and relaxation are at opposite ends of the spectrum. When you are able to maintain the balance there's a good chance of you remaining healthy and happy. However, when the scales tip and stress outweighs relaxation, symptoms of ill-health often rear their heads. With our fast pace of life and our heavy commitments, taking time out for ourselves is often a luxury we consider we cannot afford. But in reality can we afford *not* to make time to relax and unwind, for we know the powerful effect stress can have on us. It has been shown to suppress ovulation in menstruating women, to greatly contribute to digestive disorders like irritable bowel syndrome, and to play a key part in migraine headaches and depression.

The importance of relaxation

The ability to switch off and refresh ourselves is the key to sanity, but it may not be as easy as it sounds. When you are preoccupied, wound up and tense, it may be hard to lose sight of the benefits of taking time out. Being able to relax thoroughly is actually an acquired skill, which for some of us takes a little practice, but all that is required is some time, and a comfortable space in which to spend that time. Once you have learned the art of relaxation you can practise it at any time, and, best of all, it is free. Even setting aside time to *think* is therapeutic. Sometimes we go headlong into adverse situations simply because we didn't make time to plan tactics, something which is as true for family and social situations as it is for problems at work.

We all deal with the stresses and strains of life in different ways. Some of us bottle them up and then fall apart one rainy day. Others soldier on feeling disgruntled and perhaps comfort-eat or take to the bottle as a result. Regardless of how stress affects you, it is important to take some quiet time each day; as little as 15 or 20 minutes is all that is needed.

A simple technique

You will need a quiet space where you can confidently switch off. If necessary, put the answerphone on, or take the phone off the hook. Let other family members know that you don't want to be disturbed for a while, and put on some comfortable loose clothes. Either lie down on a mat, on a soft carpet or a firm bed. Make sure that you are comfortable with the room temperature and lighting. You can play some calming music in the background. Once you feel comfortable, do the following, step-by-step:

1. Place a pillow under your head, and stretch out full length. Relax your arms and your lower jaw.
2. Take a few slow deep breaths before you begin.
3. Then concentrate on relaxing your muscles, starting with the toes on one foot and then the other. Gradually work your way slowly up your body, going through all the muscle groups.
4. As you do so, first tense each group of muscles and then relax them, taking care to breathe deeply as you relax.
5. When you reach your head, and your face feels relaxed, remain in the relaxed position for 10 to 15 minutes.
6. Gradually allow yourself to 'come to'.

There are many other relaxation methods available, some with which you will be familiar. Yoga and meditation are both widely practised techniques, which allow you to practise mind over matter. Massage is a useful tool, and many of the martial arts like tai chi are therapeutic too. If you find it difficult to close your mind down, it may be a good idea to choose a system of relaxation to try and then get a little tuition in its principles. You will find some suggested further reading on page 335 and there will undoubtedly be evening classes available somewhere in your local area.

CHAPTER **20**

Your vision of health and beauty

I f you talk to six different people, you will probably find six quite different views on how to succeed in life and fulfil your dreams. Some may even suggest that there is no point to dreaming, for fate will take charge of your destiny. While each of us is perfectly entitled to our own view, there is now significant evidence to suggest that you can get much of what you wish for by applying specific techniques. Positive thinking, when channelled correctly, can go an awfully long way to getting you to where you'd like to be, in the shape that you would like to be in.

If you are completely happy with your lot, this chapter may be of little interest to you. If, however, you feel that there is room for improvement, and you are interested in achieving some of your goals, then come exploring!

The power of visualisation can help to bring good things into your life. In this chapter I would like to pass on some exceedingly useful and valuable tools that I have discovered through the works of others, which will help you to fulfil your dreams, whatever they may be.

Until two years ago I thought that the technique of visualising was a pleasant pastime, a formal way of daydreaming. In a way I was right, but I soon discovered that it was far more powerful than I had ever imagined.

The power of visioning

While on holiday a few years ago a friend lent me a book entitled *Mind Power*, by John Keyhoe, which she had been reading on the recommendation of another friend, to help find a solution to her financial problems. The book was an entertaining read about the power of visioning. As I progressed through the book I read various case histories that particularly stuck in my mind. One was about an individual who had terminal cancer and had managed to visualise the tumour away altogether, which I found incredible. The second was a story about a professional sports team in America that was split into three groups. One group trained for six weeks, one group visualised they trained for the same period of time and the final group were couch potatoes. The final fitness tests revealed that the group that had visualised their training were as fit as those that had trained. Once again I was amazed. The last story was about an old lady who was feeling lonely following the death of her husband. She attended one of John Keyhoe's workshops and learned the art of visioning, and within a short while she met an ideal suitor, whom she subsequently married. I filed the concept under intriguing in my head and got on with my life.

About a month later, after chewing it over, I decided to start visioning eating wheat with no ill-effects on my body. I'd had a severe wheat allergy for 20 years which meant I couldn't eat wheat without really suffering. I didn't dream it would work, but as it was an enjoyable pastime I continued for many months. Each morning, as I woke up, I would spend five minutes imagining my body would be completely healthy even if I ate wheat. Then in the evening, just before I went to sleep, I would imagine I was eating whatever wheat feast took my fancy. I mentally munched my way through all my old favourites, including bagels, Danish pastries and big bowls of pasta. I became so good at the process I swear I could even taste the food.

About six months later I happened to be at a wheat buffet and decided to throw caution to the wind. Once I got started I was like a human vacuum cleaner. My family looked on with horror, as they knew what would happen in the days to follow, but nothing did. I was absolutely fine, and have been ever since. It seemed like a miracle at the time, and I felt like a child at a birthday party every day for about six months afterwards.

The vision of health

Just over a year ago, after burning the candle at both ends for too long, I ended up with a major health problem, which should have required major surgery and a long recuperation period. Instead, I met up with Dr Lucia Capacchione, an American art therapist, who had cured herself of a terminal illness some years before, and she explained her methods of self-healing. I did two of Dr Capachionne's workshops that week. One on self-healing and one on visioning. Within a very short time I knew that her methods held the key not only to the resolution of my problems, but also to designing my life the way I wanted it.

I began the self-healing process, and within six weeks the consultant said that he was impressed with my progress. At my next appointment with him, six weeks later, there was no trace of my former problem, and he told me that I had defied medical science!

Designing dreams

After meeting Dr Capachione, and reading her book *Visioning*, I set about making a huge collage from magazine clippings, of all the positive things I wanted in my life. I called the collage 'The Transition', as my goal was to go from being stressed and overwhelmed, to feeling relaxed and in control. Within two weeks of making the collage, and gazing at it daily, everything started to fall into place the way I had designed it. Many other positive and wondrous things have happened to me this year, which is very uplifting.

Since starting along this path I have met people who have

had all sorts of unexpected success, including financial wind-falls that enabled them to fulfil a lifelong dream, several that found an ideal partner, and even those that received an unex-pected job offer. As a result of my own experiences, I very firmly believe that we can design life the way we want it and work towards achieving it, rather than drifting along taking what comes our way. The process of making a collage of your dreams is not only therapeutic but also a powerful tool in real-ising your goals.

Designing your vision

In her book *Visioning*, Dr Capacchione lays out a ten-step plan to designing the life of your dreams. You can wish for anything you like, within reason. It may be that you would like to find an ideal partner, or perhaps a new car which currently seems out of reach. A new home may be high on your wish list, or maybe your goal is to be slimmer and more attractive to oth-ers. You can actually wish for your heart's desire, but the first thing you will need to do is sit quietly, perhaps with some relax-ing music, and concentrate, with your eyes closed, on what it is that you desire exactly. You will need to sum up the goal or the desire in a short phrase and then write it down.

The next part of the procedure is to gather together some magazines, and armed with a pair of scissors, go through them clipping pictures and slogans that take your fancy. Dr Capacchione insists that you need to 'grab what grabs you'. In other words, clip the pictures and the words or slogans in the features and in the adverts to which you feel attracted. Stockpile your clippings until you feel you have enough mate-rial and then get ready for the editing process.

You will eventually be sticking your images and words on to a large sheet of cartridge paper, so you will need a poster sized piece of cartridge paper, some glue and some coloured pens and pencils. We usually have far too many images from the clipping phase to fit on, so editing will be necessary. While you are being so focused on the positive, you may be aware of lit-tle voices in your head telling you that this is a load of rubbish, and that you will never achieve your goals. Have a couple of pens handy, preferably of two different colours, and write down the negative messages that are going through your mind. Dr Capacchione says that it's the Critic that lives within us, and it's important to get it all out. Once the critical voice has finished having its say, you then need to reply to it with the other coloured pen, with your non-dominant hand. This hand, which is not usually used so much for writing, will allow you to work from the right side of your brain, which is the creative side, rather than from the left side, which is the rational part of the brain connected to your dominant hand. You can tell the critical voice to shove off in no uncertain terms. You don't have to be polite, you can be as rude as you like, but make yourself heard.

The next step is to edit your images and words and arrange them on your cartridge paper, which will eventually be your collage. When you have them all in position, in the way you want them, you can begin to stick them down. Make sure you are in a peaceful environment, preferably without any interruptions.

When the collage is complete have a good look at it. The messages you get from it may be quite clear, but you may need to have some dialogue with the images to ask them what they are trying to communicate to you. Once again you can ask the questions with your dominant hand and reply with the non-dominant in different coloured ink.

Put your collage in a prominent place in your home, so that you can look at it several times each day. Spend your time imagining that you have achieved your goal. If it's a new house, imagine what it will feel like to live there, getting the sensations of what it feels like to be in each room. Or if it's a new car, get the sensation of driving it, along with the admiring glances. If your goal was to be slim and attractive, indulge yourself, imagine you are and just what it feels like to be that way. Spend some time imagining the celebration that you would have to mark the achievement of the goal. These wonderful daydreams are very therapeutic, and they do actually help to turn the dreams into reality.

You can read more about Dr Capacchione's ten-step plan to designing the life of your dreams in her book *Visioning*, which is available from our mail order service, (see details on page 317). It is a lovely book, and well worth the investment.

The thought of being able to create your life the way you want it and design your dreams is so much fun. It so beats sitting waiting for things to happen to you, or just accepting what comes your way. We do run workshops from time to time, and Dr Capacchione visits the UK each year now, so if you are interested in finding out more you can contact the WNAS for details (see page 317).

The Model Diet Plan

CHAPTER **21**

The Healthy Eating Plan

Welcome to Part Three of *The Model Plan*. Now is the time to get started on your new Healthy Eating Plan. By now you will have realised the short-comings of your previous diet and should have a good idea of which foods are likely to give you the nutrients which may have previously been in short supply. The little extra time you spend planning and shopping will pay dividends in the long-term, and your new diet need not be any more expensive than your previous diet. When we worked out what the average person had previously been spending on chocolate, crisps, cola, pre-prepared food and alcohol, they almost ended up making savings by eating a more nutritious diet.

Have a read through the Healthy Eating Plan. You can make selections from the Fast Option section, or you can follow the suggested menus; in fact, you could even combine the two if you prefer. Use the Fast Options on the days when you have the least time, and on days when you are at home, or entertaining, you could prepare something a bit more sophis-ticated.

You will find weekly diaries in the Discovery Diet chapter. I suggest that you complete these for at least the first four weeks to help you get established on the Healthy Eating Plan. This involves keeping a note of everything that passes your lips, including food, snacks and drinks, and it also has space for you to note down your exercise and any supplements you have been taking. Don't cheat, as you will only be fooling yourself! Make a point of writing your diary at the same time each day so that you get into a routine, it's all too easy to forget.

The first week of the new plan may be the hardest to get through, as it is likely that you experience withdrawal symptoms, especially if you have been a regular caffeine consumer. You may get headaches, feel anxious and even feel drained of energy. Don't be put off as these feelings will pass within a few days, and certainly within a week or two you should be feeling far better than you have for some time. If you feel bad, go back and read some of the Case Histories for a bit of encouragement.

Let's start with the foods that are allowed and the things to avoid.

Food allowances and cooking instructions

Meat and fish Always use lean cuts and trim the excess fat.

Fried food Use the stir-fry method with a minimum of oil, and keep fried foods to a minimum.

Oils and fats Use polyunsaturated oils, e.g. sunflower, rape, walnut and sesame. Polyunsaturated spreads like Flora are preferable to butter. Small amounts of butter can be used on toast or crackers if preferred.

Sugar and sweet foods Keep sugar-rich foods to a minimum, and always consume after a wholesome meal. Options for cooking include fructose, concentrated apple juice and small amounts of honey.

Bread Try to incorporate a variety of grains into your diet as well as wheat, including rye, oats, corn and rice. Health food shops often stock a good variety of breads.

Bran Avoid bran and foods containing bran completely as it impedes the absorption of good nutrients.

Salt and salty foods Try not to add salt to cooking or at the table especially if fluid retention is a problem, as it tends to drag fluid into the cells. We already consume too much salt.

Fruit Preferably fresh, although tinned in fruit juice is permitted. Aim to eat three portions of fresh fruit per day (e.g. one apple, one bowl of berries or half a banana = one portion).

Vegetables Aim to consume three portions of fresh vegetables daily including one green leafy vegetable, i.e. cabbage, spinach, broccoli, kale, Brussels sprouts, etc. Where possible have raw vegetables in salads and raw vegetable crudités. Cook in the minimum amount of water, or steam if possible.

Tea and coffee Avoid caffeine and keep decaffeinated tea or coffee to a maximum of four cups per day. Ideally try some of the alternatives listed on page 30.

Milk and yoghurt Aim to consume between 400–600ml of milk per day, preferably semi-skimmed. Try to consume live yoghurt (bio yoghurt).

Cheese A variety of cheeses is permitted – a portion of 50g daily if desired.

Eggs One, preferably free-range, may be consumed daily if desired.

THE HEALTHY EATING PLAN

*= recipe provided

FAST OPTION BREAKFASTS

- Wheat- or oat-based muesli with chopped fresh fruit and semi-skimmed milk
- Wake-up muesli* with chopped fruit and semi-skimmed milk
- 2 slices of wholegrain toast with peanut butter plus a mashed banana
- Yoghurt with fresh fruit salad and nuts and seeds
- 2 slices of wholegrain toast with scrambled eggs
- 1 toasted bagel with an egg lightly fried in olive oil

- Wake-up muesli* with natural bio yoghurt, grapes and semi-skimmed milk
- Veggie sausages with baked beans, poached egg and sautéed potatoes
- 1 toasted muffin with nut butter or honey
- 2 boiled eggs with soldiers

FAST OPTION LUNCHES
- Jacket potato with tuna and salad
- Baked beans on toast
- Chicken, avocado and salad sandwich on wholegrain bread
- 'Homestyle' chicken and vegetable soup with French bread
- Omelette with a salad
- Tuna, mayonnaise and sweetcorn sandwich on wholegrain bread
- Toasted cheese and ham sandwich on ciabatta with a salad
- Tuna pasta salad
- Vegetable soup with wholegrain bread
- Jacket potato with cottage cheese and salad

FAST OPTION DINNERS
- Cold chicken or turkey salad with a jacket potato
- Grilled lamb chop with assorted vegetables
- Spaghetti bolognaise
- Chicken and cashew nut stir-fry with rice or noodles
- Poached salmon with assorted vegetables
- Goat's cheese and spinach pizza with salad
- Roasted Mediterranean vegetables with feta cheese
- Spinach and mushroom omelette
- Mixed bean chilli with rice and pitta bread
- Falafel with hommos, salad and pitta bread
- Veggie sausages with mashed potatoes, broccoli and carrots
- Quorn and vegetable stir-fry with rice or noodles
- Cauliflower and broccoli cheese* with a piece of bread

FAST OPTION DESSERTS
- Fresh fruit salad* with yoghurt

- Fruit and Yeo Valley yoghurt
- Ice-cream, banana and chopped nuts
- Apple crumble and custard or Yeo Valley crème fraîche
- Stewed apple with sultanas and cinnamon with custard

SWEET SNACKS

- Muesli bars
- Sesame seed snaps
- Flapjacks
- Wake-up snack bar
- Pancakes with Yeo Valley fruit compôte
- Wholemeal digestive biscuits
- Rice cakes with pure fruit spread
- Fruit scone
- Toast and honey or peanut butter
- Fresh fruit
- Dried fruit
- Yeo Valley yoghurt

SAVOURY SNACKS

- Cheese and crackers or oat cakes
- Cheese scone
- Rice cakes with nut butter
- Cheese and biscuits
- Poppadums with hoummos
- Kettle crisps and taramasalata or guacamole
- Japanese rice crackers
- Cheese on toast
- Toasted bagel with nut butter

BEVERAGES

- Water
- Herbal tea
- Redbush or Rooibos herbal tea look-alike
- Decaffeinated coffee (no more than 2-3 cups per day)
- Amé, Aqua Libra (lightly carbonated herbal fruit drinks)
- Fruit juice and fruit smoothies

SAMPLE MENU – 2 WEEKS

DAY 1
BREAKFAST
2 slices of wholegrain toast with peanut butter and a banana
LUNCH
Jacket potato with tuna, mayonnaise and sweetcorn plus salad
DINNER
Chicken and veggie stir-fry with rice or noodles
DESSERT
Ice-cream with banana and chopped nuts

DAY 2
BREAKFAST
Corn Flakes, a few almonds and sunflower seeds, banana
and semi-skimmed milk
LUNCH
Turkey salad sandwich on wholegrain bread
DINNER
Grilled lamb chop glazed with mustard and honey with
broccoli, carrots and mashed potato
DESSERT
Crushed meringue with fresh strawberries and Greek yoghurt

DAY 3
BREAKFAST
Bagel toasted with grilled bacon and tomatoes with
scrambled eggs
LUNCH
'Homestyle' soup with French bread and a little piece of
Edam cheese
DINNER
Grilled salmon with honey and ginger, served with salad or
broccoli, mangetout and new potatoes
DESSERT
Fresh fruit salad with natural yoghurt and few almonds

DAY 4

BREAKFAST
2 egg omelette with baked beans and toast

LUNCH
Toasted cheese and ham sandwich on ciabatta bread with salad

DINNER
Grilled chicken breast marinated in lime and coriander, served with rice and steamed vegetables

DESSERT
Fresh pineapple sprinkled with brown sugar, grilled and served with Greek yoghurt

DAY 5

BREAKFAST
Raspberry and peach yoghurt smoothie
1 bagel, toasted

LUNCH
Chicken, avocado and rocket sandwich on wholegrain bread

DINNER
Spaghetti bolognaise

DESSERT
Apple and blackberry crumble with custard or Yeo Valley crème fraîche

DAY 6

BREAKFAST
Pancakes with a chopped banana, a little pure maple syrup and chopped nuts

LUNCH
Jacket potato with baked beans and cheese

DINNER
Fish pie with cheesy mashed potato topping
Broccoli, carrots and sweetcorn

DESSERT
Ice-cream with fresh raspberries

DAY 7

BREAKFAST

Rice Krispies with a few nuts and seeds, plus a piece of fruit with semi-skimmed milk

LUNCH

Cheese or chicken ploughman's with French bread

DINNER

Bacon and mushroom omelette with goats' cheese and salad

DESSERT

Stewed apple and sultanas with ground cinnamon served with custard

DAY 8

BREAKFAST

Oat cereal or porridge with a little honey or pure maple syrup, plus a banana

LUNCH

Salmon or tuna salad with bread or a jacket potato

DINNER

Chicken cooked in tomatoes, garlic, olive oil with mushrooms and basil served with pasta or rice

DESSERT

Mixed berries served with natural yoghurt or ice-cream

DAY 9

BREAKFAST

2 boiled eggs with wholegrain soldiers

LUNCH

Grilled cherry tomatoes, courgettes, onions, garlic in olive oil with mozzarella or feta cheese with ciabatta of French bread

DINNER

Shepherd's pie with broccoli, savoy cabbage and carrots

DESSERT

Baked apple with mincemeat served with natural bio yoghurt or crème fraîche

DAY 10
BREAKFAST
Wake-up muesli* with chopped melon and semi-skimmed milk
LUNCH
Tuna and cottage cheese salad sandwich on wholegrain bread
DINNER
Chilli con carne with rice
DESSERT
Small bowl of oat crunchy cereal with semi-skimmed milk

DAY 11
BREAKFAST
2 muffins, toasted served with 2 eggs fried lightly in olive oil
LUNCH
Jacket potato with coleslaw and salad
DINNER
Lamb kebabs, brushed with garlic and mint, served with hoummos, salad and toasted pitta bread
DESSERT
Mango and strawberry smoothie

DAY 12
BREAKFAST
Fresh fruit salad with yoghurt and a few nuts and seeds
1 slice of wholegrain toast with sugar free jam (Meridian or St Dalfour)
LUNCH
Toasted tuna, mozzarella, tomato and spinach sandwich on ciabatta or French bread
DINNER
Poached cod with a cheese sauce, green beans, carrots and peas
DESSERT
Stewed plums with ginger and honey with ice-cream

DAY 13

BREAKFAST
Wake-up muesli* with grapes and strawberries, with semi-skimmed milk and bio yoghurt

LUNCH
Egg mayonnaise and salad sandwich on wholegrain bread

DINNER
Roast chicken (ready roasted from supermarket) with broccoli, carrots, peas, sweetcorn and potatoes roasted in olive oil

DESSERT
Grilled banana with cinnamon, ginger and brown sugar with yoghurt or ice-cream

DAY 14

BREAKFAST
2 slices of wholegrain toast with peanut butter and a banana

LUNCH
'Homestyle' soup with French bread

DINNER
Chicken kebabs, brushed with sesame oil, lemon juice and honey served with stir-fry vegetables and rice

DESSERT
Rice pudding with raspberries

SAMPLE VEGETARIAN MENU – 2 WEEKS

DAY 1

BREAKFAST
Scrambled eggs on wholegrain toast with baked beans and mushrooms

LUNCH
Waldorf salad with French bread

DINNER
Mushroom risotto served with ciabatta bread and a large mixed salad

DESSERT
Poached plums and ginger with custard or crème fraîche

DAY 2

BREAKFAST
Natural bio yoghurt with a banana, strawberries plus a few almonds and sunflower seeds

LUNCH
Leek and potato soup with French bread and a little goats' cheese

DINNER
Quorn bolognaise with salad, drizzled with olive oil, balsamic vinegar and lemon juice

DESSERT
Meringue filled with fresh strawberries and fromage frais

DAY 3

BREAKFAST
Wake-up muesli* or Rice Krispies with milk, a chopped pear and a few almonds

LUNCH
Cheese omelette with salad and a small chunk of wholegrain bread

DINNER
Chickpea, spinach and potato curry with rice and a poppadum

DESSERT
Rice pudding with stewed summer berries

DAY 4

BREAKFAST
Wake-up muesli* with milk and yoghurt, plus a chopped banana

LUNCH
Vegetable soup with wholegrain bread and a little piece of cheese

DINNER
Veggie sausages with mashed potatoes, broccoli and carrots

DESSERT
Small bowl of cereal with milk

DAY 5

BREAKFAST
Bagel with cream cheese and a mashed banana

LUNCH
Grilled peppers, onions and courgettes with feta cheese and ciabatta bread

DINNER
Tofu chilli with rice

DESSERT
Ice-cream with fresh strawberries

DAY 6

BREAKFAST
Muffin toasted with a poached egg and sautéed mushrooms

LUNCH
Rice, sultana and nut salad with walnut oil and balsamic vinegar dressing

DINNER
Root vegetable casserole with broccoli and green beans

DESSERT
Fresh fruit salad with yoghurt and nuts

DAY 7

BREAKFAST
Porridge with maple syrup and a few almonds

LUNCH
Tomato, basil and mozzarella on ciabatta with salad

DINNER
Falafel with hoummos, salad and pitta bread

DESSERT
Flapjack

DAY 8

BREAKFAST
Mushroom and tomato omelette

Spinach, watercress and rocket drizzled with pumpkin seed oil, balsamic vinegar, with goat's cheese and pine nuts

DINNER

Quorn and vegetable stir-fry with rice or noodles

DESSERT

Fromage frais blended with summer berries

DAY 9

BREAKFAST

Toasted muffin with nut butter or honey

LUNCH

Jacket potato with mixed beans and salad

DINNER

Tofu satay with stir-fry vegetables and rice or noodles

DESSERT

Waffles with strawberries and ice-cream

DAY 10

BREAKFAST

Veggie sausages grilled with baked beans and scrambled eggs

LUNCH

Salad with hoummos and pitta bread

DINNER

Cauliflower and broccoli cheese with a piece of bread

DESSERT

Fresh fruit salad with yoghurt and almonds

DAY 11

BREAKFAST

Wake-up muesli* with milk and a chopped banana, plus a few sunflower seeds

LUNCH

Jacket potato with goats' cheese and coleslaw

DINNER

Mixed bean chilli with rice and pitta bread

DESSERT
Grilled nectarines sprinkled with brown sugar, nuts and
cinnamon served with ice-cream or yoghurt

DAY 12
BREAKFAST
Pancakes filled with Yeo Valley summer fruit compôte with
Greek yoghurt
LUNCH
Veggie burger in a bun with a large salad
DINNER
Roasted Mediterranean vegetables with feta cheese
DESSERT
Meringue crushed with raspberries and fromage frais

DAY 13
BREAKFAST
Wake-up muesli* with milk, a chopped banana and yoghurt
LUNCH
Baked beans on toast
DINNER
Goats' cheese and spinach pizza with salad
DESSERT
Apple and blackberry crumble with custard or Yeo Valley
crème fraîche

DAY 14
BREAKFAST
2 slices of toast with nut butter
Fresh fruit
LUNCH
Greek salad with pitta bread
DINNER
Spinach and mushroom omelette with salad and jacket
potato
DESSERT
Stewed apple and pear with sultanas, cinnamon and nutmeg
served with yoghurt or ice-cream

CHAPTER **22**

The Discovery Diet – The 8-week experiment

BASIC RULES – THE FIRST FOUR WEEKS

Foods that can be eaten

In the first four weeks, during Phase One, it is very important to eat only the allowed foods. If you introduce other foods you will lose the beneficial effects of the diet and it will be necessary for you to begin again!

(* = recipe provided)

Meat and poultry

For non-vegetarians: all meat, including lamb, beef, pork, chicken, turkey, other poultry and game, and offal such as liver, kidneys, sweetbreads and hearts, can be eaten if desired. Meat and poultry can be fresh or frozen.

Meat must be lean, with all visible fat trimmed before cooking. Do not eat the skin of chicken or other poultry; it should be removed before or after cooking.

Fish and shellfish

For non-vegetarians: all types are included and they may be fresh or frozen. Do not eat the skin as it is high in fat and calories.

Note: all meat, poultry, and fish should be cooked by grilling, dry-roasting, steaming, baking, or stir-frying with low-fat ingredients, e.g. tomatoes or vegetables.

All vegetables

You can and should eat large amounts of vegetables, especially green vegetables or salad foods daily.

Root vegetables, e.g. potatoes and parsnips, are limited to one small portion per day if desired. Beans and peas, which are protein-rich vegetables, are also included in moderate amounts.

Vegetarian proteins

For vegetarians and vegans these are an essential part of the diet. You are allowed all types of nuts, beans, peas, lentils, seeds, corn-maize, rice and potatoes. Vegans in particular should have two or three portions of these per day. Some people experience abdominal bloating and wind with beans and these should be well cooked.

Fruits

All fruits are allowed, except glacé fruits and tinned fruits with sugar. Keep tinned fruits without sugar, and dried fruits to a minimum. If you want to eat bananas (the world's most popular fruit), half of one is equal to a single fruit portion. Your fruit allowance amounts to three pieces of fruit per day. Fruit can be eaten whole or as a fruit salad.

Reduced calorie foods

Fortunately, there are now many excellent calorie-reduced versions of such foods as salad dressings, mayonnaise, soups and baked beans. As a rule pre-prepared meals should be avoided on the Discovery Diet.

Vegetable oils and vegetable mayonnaise

Small amounts of these foods are allowed daily. You can have up to two teaspoons of a low-fat polyunsaturate-rich margarine, such as Flora Light, per day. There are no fried foods on the diet (you didn't really expect them, did you?), but there are some stir-fry dishes and here you just wipe the inside of the pan or wok with a piece of kitchen roll dipped in sunflower or corn oil.

Nuts and seeds

Brazil nuts, almonds, pistachios, cashews, peanuts, sunflower seeds and sesame seeds are very nutritious, but unfortunately high in calories. If you are using the Wake-up muesli* for breakfast that will be considered to be your daily allowance of nuts, seeds and dried fruit. The Wake-up sprinkle* which is also made of ground nuts and seeds is allowed on three occasions during a week to help liven up a salad or a fruit dish – see suggested menus on page 185.

Rice and other salads

White or brown rice of any variety – long grain, short grain or basmati – is allowed. It will often be used instead of potatoes. Rice bread like Bar Kat or Glutafin is available in most health food stores and some supermarkets, as are rice cakes and corn cakes. These can be used in place of bread. Additionally, buckwheat, bamboo shoots, sago and tapioca and dahl flour products, like poppadums, can be used.

Breakfast cereals

Only Cornflakes and rice cereal, and the Wake-up muesli (see page 254) are included in Phase One. They contain a good amount of protein and are often fortified with extra vitamin B and iron. Other breakfast cereals are not allowed.

Eggs

Up to seven eggs per week are allowed, unless you are known to have a very high cholesterol level. They are highly nutritious and very good value for money.

Foods to be avoided or severely limited

Wheat, oats, barley and rye, millet and bran

All foods made with these, apart from the exceptions given below, are to be avoided. This means no ordinary cakes, biscuits, puddings, pasta, pastry, pies, porridge, or breakfast cereals (apart from those mentioned above). There are some cake, biscuit and pudding recipes to be found in Chapter 23. Ordinary bread made with wheatflour is off the menu in Phase One although alternatives may be used, but even these should be limited to no more than two slices per day.

Dairy products

Milk, cream and cheese are also off the menu at this stage. Use soya milk and yoghurt or rice milk as substitutes in Phase One. Butter, or a polyunsaturated low-fat spread is allowed in very small quantities: one or two level teaspoonfuls per day. However, if you suffer with premenstrual syndrome, painful breasts, or an elevated blood cholesterol level, you should have a low-fat polyunsaturated spread instead of butter.

Foods containing milk, cream, cheese, milk solids, non-fat milk solids, lactalbumin, whey, caseinates, and lactose should be avoided. The only exception to this is polyunsaturated margarine which often contains a very small amount of milk protein, lactalbumin or whey.

Vegetarians, i.e. non-meat or fish eaters, should use soya milk fortified with calcium, and should probably consume either one egg per day or good portions of beans, peas, lentils and some nuts or seeds on most days.

Animal fats and some vegetable fats

Animal fats, some vegetable fats, hard margarine, lard, dripping and suet are out, as are palm oil and coconut oil, and foods containing them. Chemically, these vegetable oils are much more like saturated animal fats than good quality sunflower or corn oil, which are high in healthier polyunsaturates. Hard margarines, which are made from hydrogenated vegetable oils, are also off the menu.

Sugar, honey, glucose and fructose (fruit sugar)

Any food made with these should be avoided in the main. This means cakes, biscuits, most ice-cream, sweets of all kinds, chocolate and puddings. This is not as depressing as it sounds. You will find suggestions for low-calorie desserts for each evening of the diet, as well as having the option to consume either fresh fruit salad or a portion of fresh fruit.

Fruit juices are high in fructose, which weight for weight has the same calories as sucrose (ordinary sugar). If you wish to include fruit juice into your diet on a regular basis, water it down.

Alcoholic beverages

Alcohol's out initially – sorry! Don't do this diet over Christmas. Even low-calorie alcoholic drinks, though they are a great improvement, are all too high in calories. You will, however, get the chance to introduce alcohol in the long-term plan.

Yeast-rich foods

This includes any foods containing yeast extract: Marmite, Oxo, Knorr and other stock cubes, vinegar, and pickled food, chutneys, piccalilli, sauces, or condiments containing yeast extract or vinegar.

Salt

Salt should not be used in cooking or at the table. This is particularly true if you experience fluid retention or high blood pressure. Salty foods such as ham, bacon and any other salted meat should be eaten sparingly. Crisps, peanuts and many convenience dinners are not on the menu at all. If you really cannot do without the salty flavour, then use a very small amount only, or better still a potassium-rich salt substitute like LoSalt. Try flavouring any salads, vegetables, or cooked main dishes with pepper or herbs instead of salt. You should find that your taste for salt becomes less as you progress through the diet.

Caffeine and tannin

Both caffeine and tannin should be kept to an absolute minimum, or better still substituted with alternative drinks. Caffeine can be found in coffee, tea, chocolate and cola, plus some over-the-counter drugs. Tannin is usually found in tea and red wine. Try to have no more than two decaffeinated drinks per day, as these contain other chemicals, and instead use alternatives like dandelion coffee – particularly ground root rather than instant redbush tea, which is an excellent tea 'look-alike' while being caffeine-free and with very little tannin – chicory or any of the herbal teas.

Foods with additives

These cannot be avoided completely, but it is best to avoid those with some types of colouring and preservatives which can cause asthma, nettle-rash (urticaria), eczema and possibly migraine. These are:

E102	Tartrazine
E104	Quinoline Yellow
E110	Sunset Yellow FCF or Orange Yellow
E122	Carmoisine or Azorubine
E123	Amaranth
E124	Ponceau 4R or Cochineal Red A
E127	Erythrosine BS
E131	Patent Blue V
E132	Indigo Carmine or Indigotine
E142	Green S or Acid Brilliant Green BS or Lissamine Green
E151	Black PN or Brilliant Black PN
E180	Pigment Rubine or Lithol Rubine BK
E220-227	Sulphites – these may worsen asthma in very sensitive individuals.

Other colourings are not likely to cause any adverse reactions.

Suspect foods

Avoid any foods that you know do not suit you. For example, many people find some fruits, such as oranges or pineapple, too acidic. Even though they are not particularly high in calories you should avoid them. A not infrequent problem is an inability to digest beans, peas and some vegetables properly, resulting in excessive wind. Possible vegetables in this group include cabbage, cauliflower, onions and sweetcorn. At this point, trust your own knowledge and experience. After all, it is this that we want to increase, so let's not go against anything you know already. Accordingly you may have to adapt the day's menu or recipes to suit yourself.

Modifications for vegetarians

Both vegetarians and vegans should also allow peas, beans, lentils, soya milk, non-fermented soya produce, and increased amounts of nuts, seeds and rice. Suggested vegetarian menus for two weeks appear on pages 167-171.

DISCOVERY DIET

PHASE ONE – WEEKS 1-4

PHASE ONE – WEEK 1

What to expect?

You may notice during the beginning of Phase One that you experience some withdrawal symptoms as a direct result of giving up certain foods and drinks that you usually consume. These symptoms may be anything from headaches to fatigue, or even depression, and can last for anything from a few days to a week. The symptoms will pass and be replaced by an ever-increasing feeling of well-being.

The degree to which you suffer will depend on your existing diet. For example, if you are consuming lots of cups of coffee or tea, cola drinks, or refined sweet foods, you may find the first week of the diet is quite a challenge! Unfortunately there is no magic button to press that will get you through this phase completely unscathed, but cutting down gradually over a period of days or even a couple of weeks does seem to lessen the pain if you have been a heavy consumer.

It is probably best to begin the diet when you have a quiet week or two to spare without any major commitments. A word of advice to females is to begin the diet just after your period has arrived and not in the week your period is due. The reason for this it to prevent additional symptoms occurring at a time when you might be feeling premenstrual.

TIP

Never do your food shopping on an empty stomach. Plan your diet for the coming week and make a shopping list. Take the list with you and make sure you stick to it.

You will need the time to accustom yourself to your new way of eating and to get plenty of relaxation. This doesn't mean that you should take time off work; quite the opposite, as it is preferable that you remain occupied while on the diet. Just keep social arrangements that involve eating to a minimum. Then, if you feel tired or experience any withdrawal symptoms, you can go off to rest without any guilty feelings of having let others down.

After the first week or so of following the diet, with any possible withdrawal symptoms behind you, things should look up. By Week 3, you should have lost a few pounds – at least four, possibly as many as eight – and you may notice that a number of minor health problems have begun to improve. By Week 4 you should be feeling quite well; perhaps better than you have felt for some time and, with any luck, you will be a good deal nearer to your target weight. It is important to continue with Phase One until any symptoms you have been suffering like fatigue, anxiety, bowel problems or headaches, have abated. This will allow you to attribute any symptoms you experience in Phase Two to the foods you are introducing rather than your chronic health state.

PHASE ONE – WEEK I

* = recipe provided

NB: where alternative toast/bread is listed, please refer to the Healthy Shopping Options on page 302.

BREAKFASTS

- Wake-up muesli* with soya milk or rice milk or soya yoghurt
- Wake-up yoghurt shake* with 2 tablespoons of Wake-up sprinkle * blended in
- Fruit salad with Wake-up sprinkle* and soya yoghurt
- Gluten-free pancakes* with pure stewed apple and soya yoghurt
- Rice Krispies with a chopped banana and soya or rice milk
- Cornflakes with chopped almonds and soya or rice milk
- Boiled egg with rice cakes/corn crispbread or alternative soldiers
- Scrambled eggs, mushrooms and tomatoes with rice cakes/corn crispbread or alternative soldiers
- Mixed berry smoothie*

LUNCHES

- Beans on alternative toast
- Hoummos with raw vegetable crudité and corn wafers
- Jacket potato with baked beans
- Jacket potato with tuna and salad
- Mixed bean salad
- Mushroom omelette
- Scrambled or poached eggs on alternative toast
- Rice salad with fish or chicken
- Homemade or 'homestyle' fresh soup

DINNERS

- Cold meat or fish with a large salad**
- Corn pasta with Quorn or tofu in a tomato sauce with fresh herbs

- Corn tacos with mince or beans, guacamole and salsa with sweetcorn and salad
- Grilled gammon and pineapple and vegetables
- Cold chicken breast with a large salad and potato wedges or new potatoes
- Poached salmon with broccoli, carrots, sweetcorn and new potatoes
- Chicken and vegetable kebabs served with brown rice, sweetcorn and mangetout
- Prawn, chicken, Quorn or tofu stir-fry with rice noodles or brown rice

**salads should consist of lettuce, rocket, baby spinach, watercress, tomatoes, cucumber, and raw carrot. You can choose from a wide selection of salad leaves in the supermarket for convenience. Optional ingredients are peppers and spring onions according to taste.

VEGETARIAN OPTIONS
- Mixed beans in tomato sauce with brown rice
- Spinach and mushroom omelette with a large salad
- Gluten/dairy-free vegetarian sausages with baked beans and a jacket potato
- Quorn and vegetable kebabs served with brown rice, sweetcorn and mangetout
- Spanish omelette served with a large salad
- Corn spaghetti with a tomato and basil sauce with a few toasted pine nuts
- Quorn or tofu stir-fry with vegetables and brown rice or rice noodles

DESSERTS
- Stewed apple with homemade soya custard or Soya Dream
- Stewed mixed berries, strawberries, blackberries, blueberries, raspberries with soya yoghurt
- Baked apple*
- Meringue with fresh fruit salad

- Dried fruit compôte*
- Swedish Glace soya ice-cream plus sliced banana
- Fruit snow*

NB: Fresh fruit salad can be substituted for any of the above desserts.

SWEET SNACKS
- Soya yoghurt
- Soya fruit smoothie
- Dried fruit
- Wake-up snack bar
- Fresh fruit
- Sesame seed bar
- Fruit strips
- Gluten/dairy-free scone* with pure fruit spread

SAVOURY SNACKS
- Raw vegetables with hoummos
- Small amounts of unsalted nuts and seeds
- Rice cakes, corn crispbreads or Glutano crackers with sugar-free fruit spread
- Japanese rice crackers
- Kettle crisps with guacamole
- Mini poppadums with taramasalata
- Rice or corn cakes with nut butter

BEVERAGES
- Water
- Herbal tea and fruit teas
- Redbush or Rooibos herbal tea look-alike
- Decaffeinated coffee (no more than 2–3 cups per day)
- Amé, Aqua Libra (lightly carbonated herbal fruit drinks)
- Appletise
- Apple and ginger sparkling drink
- Fruit juice
- Fruit smoothies

WEEK 1 DIARY

DATE:

Please complete the diary on a daily basis and grade symptoms on a scale of 0-3

0 = NONE, 1 = MILD, 2 = MODERATE, 3 = SEVERE

Day 1

BREAKFAST .... LUNCH ....

DINNER .... SNACKS ....

EXERCISE .... SUPPLEMENTS ....

RELAXATION .... SYMPTOMS ....

REACTIONS ....

Day 2

BREAKFAST .... LUNCH ....

DINNER .... SNACKS ....

EXERCISE .... SUPPLEMENTS ....

RELAXATION .... SYMPTOMS ....

REACTIONS ....

Day 3

BREAKFAST .... LUNCH ....

DINNER .... SNACKS ....

EXERCISE .... SUPPLEMENTS ....

RELAXATION .... SYMPTOMS ....

REACTIONS ....

Day 4

BREAKFAST . . . . LUNCH . . . .

DINNER . . . . SNACKS . . . .

EXERCISE . . . . SUPPLEMENTS . . . .

RELAXATION . . . . SYMPTOMS . . . .

REACTIONS . . . .

Day 5

BREAKFAST . . . . LUNCH . . . .

DINNER . . . . SNACKS . . . .

EXERCISE . . . . SUPPLEMENTS . . . .

RELAXATION . . . . SYMPTOMS . . . .

REACTIONS . . . .

Day 6

BREAKFAST . . . . LUNCH . . . .

DINNER . . . . SNACKS . . . .

EXERCISE . . . . SUPPLEMENTS . . . .

RELAXATION . . . . SYMPTOMS . . . .

REACTIONS . . . .

Day 7

BREAKFAST . . . . LUNCH . . . .

DINNER . . . . SNACKS . . . .

EXERCISE . . . . SUPPLEMENTS . . . .

RELAXATION . . . . SYMPTOMS . . . .

REACTIONS . . . .

WEEK I MENUS

DAY I
BREAKFAST
Wake-up muesli* with chopped fresh fruit and soya milk
LUNCH
Turkey breast with salad and a jacket potato
DINNER
Grilled mackerel or sardines marinated in lemon juice and black pepper with broccoli, mangetout and carrots
DESSERT
Baked apple* with Soya Dream

DAY 2
BREAKFAST
Fresh fruit salad with Wake-up sprinkle* and soya yoghurt
LUNCH
Scrambled eggs and baked beans on alternative toast
DINNER
Grilled chicken brushed with balsamic vinegar, honey and lemon juice with brown rice, spinach and cauliflower
DESSERT
Stewed mixed berries, strawberries, blackberries, blueberries, raspberries with soya yoghurt

---

DAY 3
BREAKFAST
1 boiled egg with 2 corn crispbreads or alternative toast
LUNCH
Jacket potato with baked beans and coleslaw salad
DINNER
Prawn and vegetable stir-fry*
DESSERT
Meringue with fresh fruit salad

DAY 4

BREAKFAST
Gluten-free pancakes* with Yeo Valley fruit compôte and soya yoghurt

LUNCH
Homemade or 'homestyle' fresh soup with rice or corn cakes

DINNER
Grilled sardines with watercress, fennel and lemon salad

DESSERT
Swedish Glace soya ice-cream with sliced banana

DAY 5

BREAKFAST
Puffed rice with chopped fresh fruit and nuts and soya milk

LUNCH
Spinach and mushroom omelette with a large salad

DINNER
Chicken and vegetable kebabs served with brown rice, sweetcorn and mangetout

DESSERT
Soya rice pudding with a spoonful of pure fruit spread

DAY 6

BREAKFAST
2 poached eggs with grilled tomatoes, rice cakes and corn crispbreads

LUNCH
Beans on alternative toast with mixed green salad

DINNER
Corn tacos with mince or beans, guacamole and salsa with sweetcorn and mixed salad

DESSERT
Mixed berry smoothie*

DAY 7

BREAKFAST

Wake-up muesli* with soya milk or rice milk plus a chopped
banana

LUNCH

Raw vegetable crudité with Glutano corn crackers and
hoummos

DINNER

Poached salmon with broccoli, carrots, sweetcorn and new
potatoes

DESSERT

Fresh fruit salad with soya yoghurt and a few chopped
almonds

WEEK 2

The first week on any healthy eating plan is usually the worst,
and the Discovery Diet is no exception. Hopefully by now the
withdrawal symptoms should have gone, or at least be calming
down, and you should be feeling that there is a light at the end
of the tunnel.

Hopefully you haven't been so absorbed with sorting
yourself out and coping with the withdrawal symptoms that
you've forgotten to check whether you have lost any weight.
There are no hard and fast rules about how much weight you
lose and how fast, it really does vary. For example, just giving
up foods containing gluten, for the many individuals who have
been producing antibodies to gluten, may result in an almost
instant loss of fluid, which registers on the scales as rapid
weight loss. Other individuals may be slow and steady losers.
Either way it is important that you feel well as you go along,
once the withdrawal symptoms have passed, and continue to
satisfy the nutritional needs of your body.

If you have lost a few pounds in the first week you may be
feeling pleased, but don't expect to lose weight quickly every
week. It is far better to follow a wholesome plan and lose
weight gradually while meeting your body's nutritional needs

as, in this way, it is less likely that you will regain the weight at the end of the plan.

In order to keep your diet interesting, and prevent boredom setting in, it would be advisable to track down some special foods for this phase of the Discovery Diet. Avoiding common ingredients in your diet, particularly wheat, which is found so commonly in foods, can be difficult unless you stock up with plenty of interesting and tasty alternatives. There are several varieties of acceptable rice, soya and corn breads, plus crackers, crisp breads, pastas and flour mixes available – it is just a question of where to look and what precisely to look for. See Healthy Shopping Options on page 302 and Good Food – Where To Find It on page 307.

Being able to have toast or tasty crackers instead of constant rice cakes, and some acceptable pasta and pancakes, makes for a far more interesting and satisfying eating regime. I strongly recommend that you go on a shop crawl to check out what the different local supermarkets and health food shops have to offer. You will be surprised at the variation between shops; there may even be variation between branches of the same supermarket.

TIP

If you are short of time or lacking in energy go for fast options, which require little or no cooking. In the summer it is especially easy to consume raw vegetable crudité and mini poppadums, or corn chips, with dips like hoummos or guacamole, or a serving of roast chicken with salad, which can all be bought pre-prepared.

While you are adjusting to the Discovery Diet, it would be ideal if you could set aside some extra time for meal planning, shopping, especially for new products to introduce, and preparation of the food. As time progresses your eating routine will become second nature, although it does take a bit of adjustment initially.

PHASE ONE – WEEK 2

BREAKFASTS

- Wake-up muesli* with soya milk or rice milk
- Cornflakes with Wake-up sprinkle*, raisins and chopped nuts
- Gluten-free pancakes* with maple syrup and chopped almonds
- Cornflakes with a chopped banana and soya milk
- Scrambled eggs, grilled mushrooms and tomatoes with rice cakes
- Veggie sausages (gluten/dairy-free), grilled with mushrooms, tomatoes and rice cakes
- Alternative toast with nut butter
- Strawberry and banana smoothie

LUNCHES

- Grilled peppers, red onions, courgettes, baby plum tomatoes with balsamic vinegar and olive oil
- Chicken and apricot kebabs with salad
- Hoummos with raw vegetables and corn crackers
- Mackerel in olive oil with salad and a jacket potato
- Spinach omelette with salad
- Homemade or 'homestyle' soup with rice cakes or alternative toast

DINNERS

- Spanish rice*
- Tofu/Quorn and vegetable stir-fry with rice noodles or brown rice
- Roast chicken (skin removed) with fresh vegetables and new potatoes

- Cold chicken or turkey salad with new potatoes
- Steamed cod with broccoli, mange tout and new potatoes
- Corn tacos with mince or beans, guacamole and salsa with sweetcorn and salad
- Mushroom and herb risotto*
- Grilled salmon steak brushed with tamari sauce (wheat-free soya sauce), honey and lemon juice served with grilled courgettes, peppers and plum tomatoes
- Turkey and chickpeas with rice*
- Lamb chop with broccoli, mange tout, carrots and new potatoes

DESSERTS
- Fruit snow*
- Baked bananas with cinnamon and ginger served with soya ice-cream
- Stewed summer berries or Yeo Valley fruit compôte with soya yoghurt
- Gluten-free pancakes* with stewed plums or Yeo Valley fruit compôte and Soya Dream
- Fresh fruit salad
- Swedish Glace soya ice-cream
- Grilled nectarines sprinkled with a little brown sugar and crushed almonds

WEEK 2 MENUS

DAY I
BREAKFAST
Veggie sausages (gluten/dairy-free), grilled with mushrooms, tomatoes and rice cakes
LUNCH
Homemade or 'homestyle' soup with rice cakes or alternative toast and mixed salad

WEEK 2 DIARY

DATE:

Please complete the diary on a daily basis and grade symptoms on a scale of 0-3

0 = NONE, 1 = MILD, 2 = MODERATE, 3 = SEVERE

Day 1

BREAKFAST .... LUNCH ....

DINNER .... SNACKS ....

EXERCISE .... SUPPLEMENTS ....

RELAXATION .... SYMPTOMS ....

REACTIONS ....

Day 2

BREAKFAST .... LUNCH ....

DINNER .... SNACKS ....

EXERCISE .... SUPPLEMENTS ....

RELAXATION .... SYMPTOMS ....

REACTIONS ....

Day 3

BREAKFAST .... LUNCH ....

DINNER .... SNACKS ....

EXERCISE .... SUPPLEMENTS ....

RELAXATION .... SYMPTOMS ....

REACTIONS ....

Day 4

BREAKFAST . . . . LUNCH . . . .

DINNER . . . . SNACKS . . . .

EXERCISE . . . . SUPPLEMENTS . . . .

RELAXATION . . . . SYMPTOMS . . . .

REACTIONS . . . .

Day 5

BREAKFAST . . . . LUNCH . . . .

DINNER . . . . SNACKS . . . .

EXERCISE . . . . SUPPLEMENTS . . . .

RELAXATION . . . . SYMPTOMS . . . .

REACTIONS . . . .

Day 6

BREAKFAST . . . . LUNCH . . . .

DINNER . . . . SNACKS . . . .

EXERCISE . . . . SUPPLEMENTS . . . .

RELAXATION . . . . SYMPTOMS . . . .

REACTIONS . . . .

Day 7

BREAKFAST . . . . LUNCH . . . .

DINNER . . . . SNACKS . . . .

EXERCISE . . . . SUPPLEMENTS . . . .

RELAXATION . . . . SYMPTOMS . . . .

REACTIONS . . . .

DINNER
Steamed cod with broccoli, mange tout and new potatoes
DESSERT
Grilled nectarines sprinkled with a little brown sugar and
crushed almonds

DAY 2
BREAKFAST
Cornflakes with Wake-up sprinkle*, raisins and chopped nuts
LUNCH
Chicken and apricot kebabs with salad
DINNER
Spanish rice*
DESSERT
Fresh fruit salad

DAY 3
BREAKFAST
Gluten-free pancakes* with maple syrup and chopped
almonds
LUNCH
Mackerel in olive oil with salad and a jacket potato
DINNER
Roast chicken (skin removed) with fresh vegetables and new
potatoes
DESSERT
Fruit snow*

DAY 4
BREAKFAST
Strawberry and banana smoothie
Alternative toast with nut butter
LUNCH
hoummos with raw vegetables and corn crackers
DINNER
Grilled salmon steak brushed with tamari sauce (wheat-free

soya sauce), honey and lemon juice served with grilled
courgettes, peppers and plum tomatoes
DESSERT
Swedish Glace soya ice-cream

DAY 5
BREAKFAST
Wake-up muesli* with soya milk or rice milk
LUNCH
Grilled peppers, red onions, courgettes, baby plum tomatoes
with balsamic vinegar and olive oil
DINNER
Turkey and chickpeas and rice*
DESSERT
Baked bananas with cinnamon and ginger served with soya
ice-cream

DAY 6
BREAKFAST
Rice Krispies with a banana and a few almonds and
sunflower seeds with soya or rice milk
LUNCH
Jacket potato with baked beans and salad
DINNER
Lamb chop with broccoli, mange tout, carrots and new
potatoes
DESSERT
Soya yoghurt with mango and strawberries

DAY 7
BREAKFAST
2 poached eggs on alternative toast with grilled tomatoes
LUNCH
Rice and nut salad
DINNER
Grilled fresh tuna steak marinated in lemon juice, garlic and

tamari sauce, served with salad and new potatoes roasted in olive oil, and garlic

DESSERT

Rice pudding made with soya milk, served with pure fruit spread

WEEK 3

By now you should feel that your energy is slowly returning. Some people come to this realisation gradually, while others just wake up feeling different one day. Whichever way it occurs, retrospectively, it often feels like a great weight has been lifted from your shoulders.

Once you have your shopping sorted out and your new eating plan established, you must invest your newfound energy wisely. A regular exercise routine will pay dividends in terms of providing both increased energy and rate of weight loss. Exercising four or five times each week to the point of breathlessness will stimulate your brain chemistry, making you feel so much better, and it speeds up your metabolic rate, which increases the rate the body burns fat. Increase your pace gradually if you aren't used to exercising, remembering that it is not a competition, but instead you as an individual working to get your body into better shape.

If you haven't been very adventurous with your diet, through lack of time or motivation, make a point of introducing a few new products into your eating plan this week. Vary your snacks; perhaps prepare some wheat-free pancakes and add in some of the delicious sugar-free jams or spreads listed in Healthy Shopping Options, especially if you are experiencing cravings for sweet food.

It's normal to give lots of attention to food at the moment, especially the types of food that you are avoiding. Cravings for food, particularly the sweet variety like chocolate, are extremely common, especially in the premenstrual week. The minerals chromium and magnesium and B vitamins are all necessary for normal blood glucose control. Make a point of consuming plenty of green leafy vegetables, nuts and seeds, sweet peppers, chicken, rye and black pepper. If you feel you need some additional help take a course of Normoglycaemia, a special supplement rich in these nutrients which can be ordered from WNAS etc, see page 317.

see page 317.

TIP

Set yourself weekly achievement and weight-loss goals and line up a treat for yourself at the end of each week if you make your targets. It is very important to validate yourself for your efforts on a regular basis, rather than giving yourself a hard time because you are overweight and out of shape.

It is important to identify your personal reasons for wanting to be slimmer and feel healthier. Research shows that people who list the consequences of dieting, both positive and negative, and remind themselves of it regularly during the day, do twice as well on their diets as people who blindly follow routine dietary advice. It is a good idea to write a list of the positive and negative consequences of following the healthy eating plan, both immediate and longer-term, on an index card. You can then carry this around and refer to it prior to eating or exercising.

TIP

Eat your main meals from a small plate: a well-stocked medium-sized lunch or breakfast plate looks more satisfying than a large dinner plate only half filled.

Making the time for quiet thought and reflection is also an important aspect of the programme, especially if you spend your time rushing around after others. Regular relaxation has been shown to decrease stress levels. If you are not familiar with yoga or meditation relaxation techniques, try some creative visualisation, which is both easy and immensely enjoyable. Simply lie on the floor in a quiet room with a cushion under your head. Breathe slowly and deeply while relaxing your body from your toes upwards, remembering to relax your face and your jaw. When you feel relaxed concentrate on visualising yourself feeling slim, healthy and fit, or wander off mentally on an adventure. After 15 to 20 minutes bring your mind back to reality, and after a few minutes roll onto your side and get up slowly. Have a glass of water and notice how calm and refreshed you feel.

Give yourself a pat on the back this week. By now you should be well on your way to meeting your goals.

PHASE ONE – WEEK 3

BREAKFASTS

- Wake-up Muesli* with soya milk or rice milk
- Fresh fruit salad with soya yoghurt and 1 tbsp sunflower seeds
- Gluten-free pancakes* with stewed apple and cinnamon or Yeo Valley fruit compôte
- Dried fruit compôte* with soya yoghurt
- Banana and mixed summer berry smoothie*
- 2 poached eggs on alternative toast with some grilled mushrooms and tomatoes
- Rice Krispies plus a chopped pear with soya milk
- Rice cakes with organic nut butter or pure fruit spread

LUNCHES

- Jacket potato with baked beans
- Mushroom omelette with salad
- Poached haddock, new potatoes and salad
- Homemade vegetable soup with rice cakes
- Stir-fry baby spinach, mange tout, pepper and courgettes with brown rice
- Hard boiled egg salad with rice cakes
- Tinned sardines/mackerel and salad with rice cakes
- Soya yoghurt with a chopped banana and some nuts and seeds
- Baked beans on alternative toast

DINNERS
- Mixed bean chilli with brown rice and spinach
- Turkey bolognaise with rice noodles or corn pasta
- Grilled chicken with lemon and black pepper served with assorted vegetables
- Oven roasted Mediterranean vegetables (with chicken)
- Fresh tuna steak marinated in tamari sauce and lime served with salad
- Poached cod with spinach, broccoli, cauliflower and new potatoes
- Cold chicken, jacket potato and a large salad
- Homemade chicken and spinach curry with brown rice
- Homemade spinach, potato and chickpea curry with a poppadum
- Gluten/dairy-free veggie burgers with coleslaw, potato wedges and salad

DESSERTS
- Soya yoghurt with a few almonds and organic raisins
- Stewed apple, apricots and cinnamon with Soya Dream
- Banana and tofu cream*
- Banana and raspberry soya smoothie
- Fresh raspberries and Soya Dream
- Grilled fresh pineapple sprinkled with a little brown sugar

NB: Fresh fruit can be substituted as a dessert.

WEEK 3 MENUS

DAY 1

BREAKFAST

Gluten-free pancakes* with stewed apple and cinnamon or Yeo Valley fruit compôte

LUNCH

Jacket potato with baked beans and salad

DINNER

Grilled chicken with lemon and black pepper served with assorted vegetables

WEEK 3 DIARY

DATE:

Please complete the diary on a daily basis and grade symptoms
on a scale of 0-3

0 = NONE, 1 = MILD, 2 = MODERATE, 3 = SEVERE

Day 1

BREAKFAST . . . . LUNCH . . . .

DINNER . . . . SNACKS . . . .

EXERCISE . . . . SUPPLEMENTS . . . .

RELAXATION . . . . SYMPTOMS . . . .

REACTIONS . . . .

Day 2

BREAKFAST . . . . LUNCH . . . .

DINNER . . . . SNACKS . . . .

EXERCISE . . . . SUPPLEMENTS . . . .

RELAXATION . . . . SYMPTOMS . . . .

REACTIONS . . . .

Day 3

BREAKFAST . . . . LUNCH . . . .

DINNER . . . . SNACKS . . . .

EXERCISE . . . . SUPPLEMENTS . . . .

RELAXATION . . . . SYMPTOMS . . . .

REACTIONS . . . .

Day 4

BREAKFAST . . . . LUNCH . . . .

DINNER . . . . SNACKS . . . .

EXERCISE . . . . SUPPLEMENTS . . . .

RELAXATION . . . . SYMPTOMS . . . .

REACTIONS . . . .

Day 5

BREAKFAST . . . . LUNCH . . . .

DINNER . . . . SNACKS . . . .

EXERCISE . . . . SUPPLEMENTS . . . .

RELAXATION . . . . SYMPTOMS . . . .

REACTIONS . . . .

Day 6

BREAKFAST . . . . LUNCH . . . .

DINNER . . . . SNACKS . . . .

EXERCISE . . . . SUPPLEMENTS . . . .

RELAXATION . . . . SYMPTOMS . . . .

REACTIONS . . . .

Day 7

BREAKFAST . . . . LUNCH . . . .

DINNER . . . . SNACKS . . . .

EXERCISE . . . . SUPPLEMENTS . . . .

RELAXATION . . . . SYMPTOMS . . . .

REACTIONS . . . .

DESSERT
Banana and tofu cream*

DAY 2
BREAKFAST
2 poached eggs on alternative toast with some grilled mushrooms and tomatoes
LUNCH
Homemade or 'homestyle' vegetable soup with rice cakes
DINNER
Fresh tuna steak marinated in wheat-free tamari sauce and lime served with salad
DESSERT
Soya yoghurt with a few almonds and organic raisins

DAY 3
BREAKFAST
Wake-up muesli* with soya milk or rice milk
LUNCH
Stir-fry baby spinach, mange tout, pepper and courgettes with brown rice
DINNER
Oven roasted Mediterranean vegetables with chicken
DESSERT
Grilled fresh pineapple sprinkled with a little brown sugar

DAY 4
BREAKFAST
Banana, mixed summer berries and soya milk smoothie
LUNCH
Hard boiled egg salad with rice cakes
DINNER
Turkey bolognaise with rice noodles
DESSERT
Fresh raspberries and Soya Dream

DAY 5

BREAKFAST
Rice Krispies plus a chopped pear with soya milk

LUNCH
Tinned sardines and salad with rice cakes

DINNER
Homemade spinach, potato and chickpea curry with a poppadum

DESSERT
Fresh fruit salad with soya ice-cream or soya yoghurt

DAY 6

BREAKFAST
Rice cakes with organic nut butter/pure fruit spread
1 pot of fruit soya yoghurt

LUNCH
Jacket potato with hoummos and salad

DINNER
Homemade chicken and spinach curry with brown rice

DESSERT
Banana and mixed summer berry smoothie*

DAY 7

BREAKFAST
Fresh fruit salad with soya yoghurt, 1tbsp sunflower seeds, organic raisins, and a few almonds

LUNCH
Mushroom omelette with salad

DINNER
Gluten/dairy-free veggie burgers with coleslaw, potato wedges and salad

DESSERT
Stewed plums with ginger and soya yoghurt

WEEK 4

Your efforts should be paying dividends by now. The fourth week of The Discovery Diet is often the time when you begin to feel really well and energised. The withdrawal symptoms of the first week or two have passed, as have the effects of your old diet on your body. If you felt sluggish before you began, or experienced a variety of common symptoms including headaches, mood swings or bowel problems, you should notice a general improvement. For persistent, or severe to moderate symptoms, diet alone may not be sufficient. You may need the help of some specialist supplements to restore the nutrient balance in your body.

In the UK, the commonest deficiencies are of iron and vitamin B. A mild deficiency detected by blood test may not matter if the diet is well-balanced and you feel healthy. However, if symptoms or signs of deficiency are present, then corrective action will be needed.

The signs of iron deficiency are a sore tongue, recurrent mouth ulcers, cracking at the corners of the mouth, flattening of the normal curve of the finger or thumb nails, fatigue, and a pale complexion due to anaemia. A supplement of iron may well be needed as well as possible tests to determine the cause of the deficiency.

Lack of vitamin B can also produce a variety of symptoms and signs, some of which are similar to iron deficiency. They include redness or greasiness at the side of the nose, cracking at the outer corners of the eyes, or at the corners of the mouth, a sore tongue, recurrent mouth ulcers, and cracking or peeling of the lips. Furthermore, a lack of either iron or vitamin B deficiency is sometimes the cause of depression, anxiety or insomnia.

Our own research has shown the mineral magnesium to be the most common deficiency amongst women of childbearing age, with over 50 per cent suffering low levels. There are no physical signs of magnesium deficiency unfortunately, but low levels often result in muscle cramps, depression, mood changes, loss of appetite, nausea and apathy.

You can find out more about what your nutritional status is by completing the assessing nutrient levels questionnaire on page 44.

Your score will give some idea as to the likelihood of having a deficiency of vitamins or minerals. If there is a deficiency it is important that it is corrected by appropriate nutritional supplements as well as a good diet. You can find out what scientifically-based supplements have to offer in Chapter 5.

If you need to lose more than 10 pounds in weight but are otherwise in good health you are probably well advised to take a low-dose multivitamin and multi-mineral supplement.

On the whole if you are reasonably well and do not have nutritionally related problems then you could probably manage without supplements. If in doubt, an ordinary but comprehensive multivitamin (with iron if you have heavy periods) is probably the best.

It is important to remember that there is no special supplement of vitamins, minerals, or anything else for that matter, which will melt your excess weight away. There is no substitute for a well-balanced carefully selected diet, taking care to have an adequate intake of essential nutrients.

TIP

During your fourth week on the Discovery Diet you may find that your metabolic rate slows down as your body becomes used to the new way of eating and the reduced calorie intake. An excellent way of speeding up the metabolic rate is to exercise four or five times each week to the point of breathlessness. You can choose any exercise you like, from brisk walking, a formal workout, swimming, racquet sports or even just dancing to your favourite music. Apart from helping to burn up the fat and tone your body, regular exercise results in an incredible sense of well-being and as an added bonus promotes long-term health.

Rather than shopping once a week for all your food, it is preferable to shop at least twice each week, especially for fruit, vegetables and salad stuff, as the shelf-life of the vitamins and minerals in them is quite short. Make sure you store fresh produce in the refrigerator or somewhere very cool, to prevent it from spoiling.

PHASE ONE – WEEK 4
BREAKFASTS
- Wake-up muesli* with soya milk or rice milk
- Rice Krispies with raisins and chopped nuts
- Gluten-free pancakes* with stewed mixed berries or Yeo Valley fruit compôte
- Rice flakes and organic raisins soaked overnight in soya milk/apple juice with grated ginger, apple and cinnamon
- Cornflakes with a chopped banana and soya milk
- Scrambled eggs, grilled mushrooms and tomatoes with rice cakes
- Alternative toast with pure fruit spread
- Tropical mango smoothie*

LUNCHES
- Grilled peppers, red onions, courgettes, baby plum tomatoes with balsamic vinegar and olive oil
- Scrambled eggs on alternative toast
- Chicken kebabs with salad
- Jacket potato with hoummos and salad
- Grilled sardines with lemon juice, garlic and black pepper with salad
- Spinach omelette with salad
- Homemade or 'homestyle' soup with rice cakes or alternative toast
- Prawns marinated in lime, coriander and black pepper with salad

DINNERS

- Steamed salmon with broccoli, mangetout and new potatoes
- Spanish rice*
- Tofu/chicken and vegetable stir-fry with rice noodles or brown rice
- Spanish omelette* with salad
- Roast chicken (skin removed) with fresh vegetables
- Cold chicken or ham salad with new potatoes
- Turkey, sweet potato and spinach curry with brown rice
- Corn tacos with mince or beans, guacamole and salsa with sweetcorn and salad
- Hard boiled egg salad with a jacket potato
- Grilled salmon steak brushed with tamari sauce (wheat free soya sauce), honey and lemon juice served with grilled courgettes, peppers and plum tomatoes
- Turkey and chickpeas* with rice

DESSERTS

- Fruit snow*
- Baked bananas with cinnamon and ginger served with soya ice-cream
- Stewed summer berries with soya yoghurt
- Gluten free pancakes* with pure fruit spread or Yeo Valley Fruit Compôte and Soya Dream
- Fresh fruit salad
- Swedish Glace soya ice-cream
- Grilled nectarines sprinkled with a little brown sugar and crushed almonds
- Stewed apples and blackberries with soya custard

NB: Fresh fruit can be substituted as a dessert

WEEK 4 DIARY

DATE:

Please complete the diary on a daily basis and grade symptoms on a scale of 0-3

0 = NONE, 1 = MILD, 2 = MODERATE, 3 = SEVERE

Day 1

BREAKFAST .... LUNCH ....

DINNER .... SNACKS ....

EXERCISE .... SUPPLEMENTS ....

RELAXATION .... SYMPTOMS ....

REACTIONS ....

Day 2

BREAKFAST .... LUNCH ....

DINNER .... SNACKS ....

EXERCISE .... SUPPLEMENTS ....

RELAXATION .... SYMPTOMS ....

REACTIONS ....

Day 3

BREAKFAST .... LUNCH ....

DINNER .... SNACKS ....

EXERCISE .... SUPPLEMENTS ....

RELAXATION .... SYMPTOMS ....

REACTIONS ....

Day 4

BREAKFAST . . . . LUNCH . . . .

DINNER . . . . SNACKS . . . .

EXERCISE . . . . SUPPLEMENTS . . . .

RELAXATION . . . . SYMPTOMS . . . .

REACTIONS . . . .

Day 5

BREAKFAST . . . . LUNCH . . . .

DINNER . . . . SNACKS . . . .

EXERCISE . . . . SUPPLEMENTS . . . .

RELAXATION . . . . SYMPTOMS . . . .

REACTIONS . . . .

Day 6

BREAKFAST . . . . LUNCH . . . .

DINNER . . . . SNACKS . . . .

EXERCISE . . . . SUPPLEMENTS . . . .

RELAXATION . . . . SYMPTOMS . . . .

REACTIONS . . . .

Day 7

BREAKFAST . . . . LUNCH . . . .

DINNER . . . . SNACKS . . . .

EXERCISE . . . . SUPPLEMENTS . . . .

RELAXATION . . . . SYMPTOMS . . . .

REACTIONS . . . .

WEEK 4 MENUS

DAY 1
BREAKFAST
Cornflakes with a chopped banana and soya milk
LUNCH
Turkey kebabs with salad
DINNER
Corn tacos with mince or beans, guacamole and salsa with sweetcorn and salad
DESSERT
Stewed summer berries with soya yoghurt

DAY 2
BREAKFAST
Mango and banana smoothie*
2 rice cakes with nut butter
LUNCH
Grilled sardines with lemon juice, garlic and black pepper with salad
DINNER
Roast chicken (skin removed) with fresh vegetables
DESSERT
Fruit snow*

DAY 3
BREAKFAST
Rice flakes and organic raisins soaked overnight in soya milk/apple juice with grated ginger, apple and cinnamon
LUNCH
Jacket potato with hommos and salad
DINNER
Grilled salmon steak brushed with tamari sauce (wheat-free soya sauce), honey and lemon juice served with grilled courgettes, peppers and plum tomatoes

DESSERT
Fresh fruit salad

DAY 4
BREAKFAST
Wake-up muesli* with soya milk or rice milk
LUNCH
Homemade or 'homestyle' soup with alternative bread or
rice/corn cakes
DINNER
Turkey, sweet potato and spinach curry with brown rice
DESSERT
Baked bananas with cinnamon and ginger served with soya
ice-cream

DAY 5
BREAKFAST
Alternative toast with pure fruit spread
LUNCH
Spinach omelette with salad
DINNER
Tofu/chicken and vegetable stir-fry with rice noodles or
brown rice
DESSERT
Swedish Glace soya ice-cream

DAY 6
BREAKFAST
Gluten-free pancakes* with stewed mixed summer berries
LUNCH
Prawns marinated in lime, coriander and black pepper with
salad
DINNER
Spanish rice*
DESSERT
Stewed summer berries with soya yoghurt

DAY 7

BREAKFAST

Scrambled eggs, grilled mushrooms and tomatoes with rice cakes

LUNCH

Grilled peppers, red onions, courgettes, plum tomatoes with balsamic vinegar and olive oil

DINNER

Chicken or tuna salad with a jacket potato

DESSERT

Stewed apples and blackberries with soya custard or soya yoghurt

PHASE ONE – 2 WEEKS OF VEGETARIAN MENUS

DAY 1

BREAKFAST

Wake-up muesli* with chopped fresh fruit and soya milk

LUNCH

Mixed bean salad

DINNER

Quorn and vegetable kebabs served with brown rice, sweetcorn and mangetout

DESSERT

Fruit snow*

DAY 2

BREAKFAST

2 slices of alternative toast with organic nut butter

LUNCH

Homemade or 'homestyle' fresh soup with salad

DINNER

Vegetable and tofu curry with rice and spinach

DESSERT

Fresh fruit salad

DAY 3

BREAKFAST

Soya yoghurt with chopped almonds, pine nuts, a few raisins and a slice of chopped melon

LUNCH

Hoummos, raw crudité, corn chips and a large salad

DINNER

Spinach and mushroom omelette with broccoli, carrots and new potatoes

DESSERT

Stewed apple and blackberries with homemade soya custard or soya yoghurt

DAY 4

BREAKFAST

Wake-up fruit shake* with 2 tablespoons of Wake-up sprinkle* blended in

LUNCH

Jacket potato with baked beans and a side salad

DINNER

Corn spaghetti with a tomato and basil sauce with a few toasted pine nuts

DESSERT

Fresh strawberries or sliced banana and a little Soya Dream

DAY 5

BREAKFAST

Cornflakes with almonds and sultanas with soya milk

LUNCH

Scrambled or poached eggs on alternative toast

DINNER

Mixed beans in tomato sauce served with spinach, sweetcorn and brown rice

DESSERT

Soya yoghurt with a few sunflower seeds and a chopped pear

DAY 6

BREAKFAST
Boiled egg with grilled tomatoes and mushrooms and 2 alternative crackers or alternative soldiers

LUNCH
Grilled Mediterranean vegetables (peppers, courgettes, red onions, aubergine, garlic) marinated in balsamic vinegar, olive oil and lemon juice

DINNER
Gluten/dairy-free veggie sausages with new potatoes, broccoli, cauliflower and carrots

DESSERT
Gluten-free scone with pure fruit spread

DAY 7

BREAKFAST
Gluten-free pancakes with fruit compôte* filling and soya yoghurt

LUNCH
Jacket potato with hummos, chopped avocado and a large salad

DINNER
Quorn or tofu stir-fry with vegetables brown rice or rice noodles

DESSERT
Swedish Glace soya ice-cream with stewed berries

DAY 8

BREAKFAST
Wake-up fruit shake*
2 slices gluten-free toast with pure fruit spread

LUNCH
Spinach and sweet potato omelette with salad

DINNER
Quorn chilli with brown rice and tomato salsa

DESSERT
Dried fruit compôte*

DAY 9
BREAKFAST
Wake-up muesli* with soya or rice milk and chopped fresh fruit
LUNCH
Homemade or 'homestyle' leek and potato soup with rice cakes
DINNER
Vegetarian gluten/dairy-free cutlet with fresh vegetables and new potatoes
DESSERT
Raspberry, mango and coconut milk soya smoothie

DAY 10
BREAKFAST
Cornflakes with Wake-up sprinkle*, a chopped banana and soya or rice milk
LUNCH
Pear and walnut salad with walnut oil and balsamic vinegar dressing
DINNER
Gluten free/dairy-free tofu burgers with mashed potatoes and baked beans
DESSERT
Summer berries or Yeo Valley fruit compôte with soya yoghurt and a few almonds

---

DAY 11
BREAKFAST
Gluten-free pancakes with maple syrup, a banana and chopped nuts
LUNCH
Jacket potato with hoummos and a large salad

DINNER
Mushroom and herb risotto* with mangetout and baby sweetcorn
DESSERT
Baked apple* with Soya Dream

DAY 12
BREAKFAST
Dried fruit compôte with Wake-up sprinkle* and soya yoghurt
LUNCH
Stir-fried baby spinach with garlic and mushrooms served with brown rice
DINNER
Stuffed peppers* with salad
DESSERT
Banana tofu cream*

DAY 13
BREAKFAST
Mixed berry smoothie*
2 slices alternative toast with fruit spread
LUNCH
Grilled peppers, courgettes and tomatoes drizzled with balsamic vinegar, lemon juice and olive oil, served warm with salad and pine nuts
DINNER
Tomato and basil sauce with pine nuts and corn pasta
DESSERT
Grilled pineapple sprinkled with brown sugar and lemon juice

DAY 14
BREAKFAST
Scrambled eggs, mushrooms and tomatoes with rice cakes, corn crispbread or alternative soldiers

LUNCH

Stir fried tofu with a large salad plus Wake-up sprinkle*

DINNER

Corn tacos with mixed spicy beans, guacamole and salsa
with sweetcorn and salad

DESSERT

Soya yoghurt with fresh fruit and a few nuts and seeds

PHASE TWO – WEEKS 5-8

WEEK 5

Congratulations on completing Phase One of the Discovery
Diet. By now, if you have managed to stick to the plan, you
should be feeling lighter, more toned, aware of muscles you had
forgotten you had and enjoying much more energy. If you have
fallen by the wayside in the last week or so, instead of beating
yourself up mentally, simply repeat another two weeks of Phase
One, before moving on to Phase Two.

During Phase Two we will be introducing food groups one
by one to see how your body reacts. Once you have cleared your
system during Phase One you should find that your body will
become amazingly good at helping you to identify the things it
likes and dislikes. It communicates via signs and symptoms, in
this way allowing you to become a 'nutritional detective'. Very
often, when the immune system is impaired and the body reacts
to certain foods or drinks, the chemicals produced may make
you feel unwell in some way. The symptoms can vary from a
headache, even a full-blown migraine, to eczema, nettle rash
(urticaria), rhinitis, asthma, abdominal bloating and discomfort,
constipation, diarrhoea, wind, anxiety, irritability, insomnia, and
possibly premenstrual tension, panic attacks, or even feelings of
total exhaustion. The reaction may even push your weight back
up, which gives you an instant clue that all is not well.

During Week 5 of the plan, which is the first week of Phase
Two, I have put dairy products back on the menu, beginning with
milk, followed by yoghurt, then cheese and butter. You will need

to introduce only one variety of a dairy product at a time over a period of a few days, to enable your body to report back to you. If you introduce several types in quick succession you will only end up getting confused, and have to begin the process again.

If and when you do have a reaction to individual food groups, you may feel that you have had a setback, as you feel less well and may even gain some weight. Any reaction should be regarded as a positive step. It means that you have discovered some foods that don't really suit your body at the moment. A reaction, should it occur, may range from mild to severe, but is not likely to last for more than a few days and will gradually wear off. If you do experience a reaction, you will need to stop eating the suspect foods for now.

If you have reached your target weight you can proceed to Phase Two during the coming week. If you would still like to lose more weight you have the choice of repeating another two weeks of Phase One or progressing to Phase Two, knowing you may put a few pounds back on if you hit on a suspect food. Whatever you do, don't forget to fill in your diary each day.

TIP

Aim to make your main mealtime sacred so that you can enjoy your food. Eat with other family members or friends instead of eating in front of the television, and relax as you eat, chewing your food slowly while enjoying the flavours.

PHASE TWO – WEEK 5

DAIRY TRIAL
*= recipe provided
BREAKFASTS
- Cornflakes with chopped fruit and nuts and semi-skimmed milk
- Wake-up muesli* with natural bio yoghurt and semi-skimmed milk

- Wake-up fruit shake* with 2 tablespoons of Wake-up sprinkle* blended in
- Rice flakes soaked overnight in semi-skimmed milk served with stewed fruit compôte
- Gluten-free bread toasted with scrambled eggs and grilled mushrooms
- Natural bio yoghurt with fresh fruit and unsalted nuts and seeds
- Cornflakes with semi-skimmed milk, a handful of raisins and a few sunflower seeds

LUNCHES
- Cheese and spinach omelette with salad
- Greek salad (feta cheese, cucumber, red onions, beef tomatoes, salad leaves)
- Homemade or 'homestyle' soup
- Cheese salad, e.g. Edam, Cheddar, cottage cheese
- Falafel with hoummos and salad
- Jacket potato with cottage cheese and salad
- Tinned mackerel in tomato sauce with salad consisting of baby spinach and watercress
- Rice cakes with cottage cheese or Edam and salad
- Goats' cheese grilled with cherry tomatoes and courgettes served with salad
- Mozzarella, basil and tomato salad with an olive oil and balsamic vinegar dressing

DINNERS
- Hard-boiled egg and grated cheese salad
- Lamb steak, chips and salad
- Oven roasted Mediterranean vegetables with feta cheese
- Fresh grilled mackerel marinated in lemon juice and black pepper served with brown rice and salad
- Vegetable stir-fry with halloumi cheese
- Poached cod with a white sauce and steamed broccoli, spinach and new potatoes
- Spanish omelette with goats' cheese and potato wedges

- Chicken breast brushed with pesto served with a salad and jacket potato
- Cauliflower and broccoli cheese*

DESSERTS
- Blackberries with hazelnut cheese
- Rice pudding with mixed berries or Yeo Valley fruit compôte
- Natural bio yoghurt with stewed fruit
- Stewed rhubarb with custard or crème fraîche
- Ice-cream and fruit salad
- Soaked brown rice flakes in semi-skimmed milk with ground cinnamon and ginger
- Frozen yoghurt ice-cream* with sliced melon

SWEET SNACKS
- Bio fruit yoghurt
- Fresh fruit
- Cottage cheese, fresh pineapple and a few sunflower seeds
- Fruit smoothie
- Wake-up snack bar
- Sesame seed snack bars
- Fruit and nuts bars
- Fruit strips

SAVOURY SNACKS
- Small amounts of low fat cheese with rice cakes or alternative toast
- Unsalted nuts and seeds
- Small piece of cheese with an apple
- Kettle crisps with hoummos
- Mini poppadums with guacamole
- Gluten-free cheese scone*

BEVERAGES
- Water
- Herbal tea and fruit teas

- Redbush or Rooibos herbal tea look-alike
- Decaffeinated coffee (no more than 2–3 cups per day)
- Barley Cup, Caro, NoCaf
- Amé, Aqua Libra (lightly carbonated herbal fruit drinks)
- Appletise
- Apple and ginger sparkling drink
- Fruit juice
- Fruit smoothies*

WEEK 5 MENUS

DAY 1
BREAKFAST
Yoghurt shake* with 2 rice cakes and peanut butter
LUNCH
Jacket potato with hoummos and salad
DINNER
Lamb steak, chips and salad
DESSERT
Natural bio yoghurt with stewed fruit

DAY 2
BREAKFAST
Natural bio yoghurt with fresh fruit and unsalted nuts and seeds
LUNCH
Homemade or 'homestyle' soup with alternative bread and mixed salad
DINNER
Poached cod with herbs and steamed broccoli, spinach and new potatoes
DESSERT
Fresh fruit salad with ice-cream or crème fraîche and a few almonds and sunflower seeds

WEEK 5 DIARY

DATE:

Please complete the diary on a daily basis and grade symptoms on a scale of 0-3

0 = NONE, 1 = MILD, 2 = MODERATE, 3 = SEVERE

Day 1

BREAKFAST . . . . LUNCH . . . .

DINNER . . . . SNACKS . . . .

EXERCISE . . . . SUPPLEMENTS . . . .

RELAXATION . . . . SYMPTOMS . . . .

REACTIONS . . . .

Day 2

BREAKFAST . . . . LUNCH . . . .

DINNER . . . . SNACKS . . . .

EXERCISE . . . . SUPPLEMENTS . . . .

RELAXATION . . . . SYMPTOMS . . . .

REACTIONS . . . .

Day 3

BREAKFAST . . . . LUNCH . . . .

DINNER . . . . SNACKS . . . .

EXERCISE . . . . SUPPLEMENTS . . . .

RELAXATION . . . . SYMPTOMS . . . .

REACTIONS . . . .

Day 4

BREAKFAST . . . . LUNCH . . . .

DINNER . . . . SNACKS . . . .

EXERCISE . . . . SUPPLEMENTS . . . .

RELAXATION . . . . SYMPTOMS . . . .

REACTIONS . . . .

Day 5

BREAKFAST . . . . LUNCH . . . .

DINNER . . . . SNACKS . . . .

EXERCISE . . . . SUPPLEMENTS . . . .

RELAXATION . . . . SYMPTOMS . . . .

REACTIONS . . . .

Day 6

BREAKFAST . . . . LUNCH . . . .

DINNER . . . . SNACKS . . . .

EXERCISE . . . . SUPPLEMENTS . . . .

RELAXATION . . . . SYMPTOMS . . . .

REACTIONS . . . .

Day 7

BREAKFAST . . . . LUNCH . . . .

DINNER . . . . SNACKS . . . .

EXERCISE . . . . SUPPLEMENTS . . . .

RELAXATION . . . . SYMPTOMS . . . .

REACTIONS . . . .

DAY 3

BREAKFAST
Cornflakes with semi-skimmed milk, a handful of raisins and a few sunflower seeds

LUNCH
Falafel with hoummos, guacamole, tomato salsa and salad

DINNER
Chicken breast marinated in yoghurt and spices served with a jacket potato, mangetout and sweetcorn

DESSERT
Stewed rhubarb and cinnamon with custard or crème fraîche

DAY 4

BREAKFAST
Wake-up muesli* with natural bio yoghurt and semi-skimmed milk

LUNCH
Cheese and spinach omelette with salad

DINNER
Vegetable stir-fry with halloumi cheese

DESSERT
Banana and raspberry smoothie made with semi-skimmed milk and bio yoghurt

DAY 5

BREAKFAST
Scrambled eggs on alternative toast with a little butter

LUNCH
Goats' cheese grilled with cherry tomatoes served with salad

DINNER
Fresh grilled mackerel marinated in lemon juice and black pepper served with brown rice and salad

DESSERT
Blackberries with hazelnut cheese

DAY 6

BREAKFAST
Wake-up muesli* with chopped fresh fruit, natural bio
yoghurt or semi-skimmed milk

LUNCH
Jacket potato with cold turkey and a large salad

DINNER
Cauliflower and broccoli cheese

DESSERT
Frozen yoghurt*

DAY 7

BREAKFAST
Mushroom and cheese omelette with alternative toast with a
little butter

LUNCH
Falafel with hoummos and salad and a few rice cakes

DINNER
Oven roasted Mediterranean vegetables (and chicken) with
feta cheese

DESSERT
Rice pudding with summer berries or Yeo Valley fruit
compôte

Note: If you don't feel so well on dairy foods, wait a few days
before trying oats and rye.

WEEK 6

Week 5 should have revealed whether dairy products suit your
system right now. If you had no adverse reactions to any of the
dairy products you can continue to include them in your menu.
If you are unsure, look over your diaries and check to see how
you felt on the individual dairy foods and drinks. In order to
maintain your feeling of well-being it is better to continue only
with those foods that made you feel good. If you did develop
symptoms including diarrhoea, catarrh, skin irritation, weight

gain or a loss of energy, you should ideally continue to exclude these foods, and try them again during the Grand Review.

Through the coming week you will be introducing the whole grains oats and rye, and the same rules apply. Introduce each food gradually, keeping detailed notes, and weigh yourself at least every few days to see whether you gain any of the lost pounds. There is a variety of foods to try. The oat-based foods include oat cakes, porridge oats, oat crunchy cereals and oat milk. The rye foods consist of rye crackers like Ryvita (look at the labels as some contain wheat flour), Finn Crisp, pure rye bread (Village Bakery make a good rye bread which is available from supermarkets and health food shops), Pumpernickel, the flat German rye bread, and rye flour.

Begin with one of the grains only, either oats or rye, and don't move on to the next grain until you have decided whether your body wants to continue with the grain with which you have just experimented. If you get a positive reaction you can continue to include this grain into your menu, but if not leave it to one side until you reach the Grand Review (see page 249).

These grains can sometimes produce gut symptoms, ranging from indigestion to bloating and constipation. They can also affect your mood, make you feel anxious and cause a downturn in energy levels, as well as causing weight gain if they produce an antibody reaction within the body. Keep careful diary entries and watch out for these symptoms. You may be fine with both types of whole grain, only one type, or neither. It is simply a question of trying them out to determine the result.

TIP

It is important not to change any other aspect of your diet and lifestyle while you are trying these new foods, for if you do experience a reaction you need to know for certain that there was no other cause.

You should by now be noticing the difference those lost pounds make. Your clothes that were previously fit to burst should feel looser, and your body should be beginning to feel toned. It is important at this point to review your long-term goals and write down your targets. Ensure your targets are realistic and span an adequate amount of time, bearing in mind that weight loss on any healthy eating plan tends to slow down as time goes on.

TIP

By now you should have got the hang of reading your body's messages. You have done well to have got this far so why not treat yourself to a new outfit to show off your new shape?

PHASE TWO – WEEK 6

OATS AND RYE TRIAL
BREAKFAST

- Oat crunchy cereal with chopped fruit and nuts with semi-skimmed yoghurt
- Porridge made with semi-skimmed milk served with stewed fruit or Yeo Valley fruit compôte
- Wake-up muesli* with a chopped banana, with semi-skimmed milk
- Banana and mango fruit smoothie made with semi-skimmed milk and natural bio yoghurt
- Wake-up yoghurt shake*, plus 2 Ryvita with pure fruit spread
- 100% pure rye bread toasted with 2 poached or boiled eggs
- Oat cakes or Ryvita with pure fruit spread or nut (almond, cashew, peanut) butter
- 2 egg mushroom omelette with 100% pure rye bread

LUNCHES

- Rye bread sandwiches with fish, poultry, cheese or egg filling
- Homemade or 'homestyle' soup with rye bread or oat cakes

- Jacket potato with hoummos and salad
- Sardines in olive oil with a salad and oat cakes
- Scrambled eggs on 100% rye bread toast
- Natural bio yoghurt with chopped fresh fruit and nuts and seeds
- Oven roasted Mediterranean vegetables with feta cheese
- Spinach and sweet potato omelette served with salad
- Falafel with hoummos on open rye bread sandwiches
- Ryvita with cottage cheese, fresh pineapple and a few sunflower seeds

DINNER
- Tuna steak marinated in lemon juice, garlic and black pepper, grilled and served with broccoli, mangetout and new potatoes
- Stir-fry chicken or prawns and vegetables served with brown rice or rice noodles
- Pilchards in tomato sauce with salad and a jacket potato
- Oaty vegetable crumble
- Chicken breast brushed with pesto, grilled and served with fresh vegetables
- Cauliflower and broccoli cheese*
- Lamb kebabs*
- Ratatouille with brown rice and a little grated cheese
- Salmon and broccoli quiche (pastry made with rye flour) with salad
- Roasted veggie quiche (pastry made with rye flour) with salad

DESSERTS
- Tropical crumble*
- Oats soaked in semi-skimmed milk, served with bio yoghurt, stewed apple and a little pure maple syrup
- Rye pancakes with fresh fruit and bio yoghurt
- Grilled fresh pineapple sprinkled with a little brown sugar, cinnamon and lemon juice served with natural bio yoghurt
- Bio yoghurt with chopped fresh fruit and Wake-up sprinkle*

- Fresh fruit salad with yoghurt

SWEET SNACKS
- Crunchy oat cereal bar
- Bio fruit yoghurt
- Fresh fruit
- Wake-up bar
- Cottage cheese, fresh pineapple and a few sunflower seeds
- Fruit smoothie
- Sesame seed snack bars
- Fruit and nuts bars
- Fruit strips

SAVOURY SNACKS
- Rye bread with a little portion of cheese
- Oat cakes with nut butter or honey
- Small amounts of low fat cheese with rice cakes or alternative toast
- Unsalted nuts and seeds
- Small piece of cheese with an apple
- Kettle crisps with hommmos
- Mini poppadums with guacamole
- Wheat-free cheese scone*

WEEK 6 MENUS

DAY I
BREAKFAST
Oat crunchy cereal with chopped fresh fruit, nuts and semi-skimmed milk or soya milk
LUNCH
Jacket potato with hommmos and salad
DINNER
Tuna steak marinated in lemon juice, garlic and black pepper, grilled served with broccoli, mangetout and new potatoes

WEEK 6 DIARY

DATE:

Please complete the diary on a daily basis and grade symptoms on a scale of 0-3

0 = NONE, 1 = MILD, 2 = MODERATE, 3 = SEVERE

Day 1

BREAKFAST .... LUNCH ....

DINNER .... SNACKS ....

EXERCISE .... SUPPLEMENTS ....

RELAXATION .... SYMPTOMS ....

REACTIONS ....

Day 2

BREAKFAST .... LUNCH ....

DINNER .... SNACKS ....

EXERCISE .... SUPPLEMENTS ....

RELAXATION .... SYMPTOMS ....

REACTIONS ....

Day 3

BREAKFAST .... LUNCH ....

DINNER .... SNACKS ....

EXERCISE .... SUPPLEMENTS ....

RELAXATION .... SYMPTOMS ....

REACTIONS ....

Day 4

BREAKFAST . . . . LUNCH . . . .

DINNER . . . . SNACKS . . . .

EXERCISE . . . . SUPPLEMENTS . . . .

RELAXATION . . . . SYMPTOMS . . . .

REACTIONS . . . .

Day 5

BREAKFAST . . . . LUNCH . . . .

DINNER . . . . SNACKS . . . .

EXERCISE . . . . SUPPLEMENTS . . . .

RELAXATION . . . . SYMPTOMS . . . .

REACTIONS . . . .

Day 6

BREAKFAST . . . . LUNCH . . . .

DINNER . . . . SNACKS . . . .

EXERCISE . . . . SUPPLEMENTS . . . .

RELAXATION . . . . SYMPTOMS . . . .

REACTIONS . . . .

Day 7

BREAKFAST . . . . LUNCH . . . .

DINNER . . . . SNACKS . . . .

EXERCISE . . . . SUPPLEMENTS . . . .

RELAXATION . . . . SYMPTOMS . . . .

REACTIONS . . . .

DESSERT

Grilled fresh pineapple sprinkled with a little brown sugar, cinnamon and lemon juice served with natural bio yoghurt

---

DAY 2

BREAKFAST

Wake-up muesli* with a chopped banana, with semi-skimmed milk

LUNCH

Sardines in olive oil with a salad and oat cakes

DINNER

Chicken breast brushed with pesto sauce, grilled and served with fresh vegetables

DESSERT

Bio yoghurt with chopped fresh fruit and Wake-up sprinkle*

DAY 3

BREAKFAST

Banana and mango fruit smoothie made with semi-skimmed milk or soya milk
2 oatcakes with pure fruit spread

LUNCH

Oven roasted vegetables with feta cheese

DINNER

Oaty vegetable crumble

DESSERT

Rice pudding served with puréed summer berries or Yeo Valley fruit compôte

---

DAY 4

BREAKFAST

Porridge made with semi-skimmed milk served with stewed fruit

LUNCH

Spinach and sweet potato omelette served with salad

DINNER

Stir-fry chicken or prawns and vegetables served with brown rice or rice noodles

DESSERT

Fresh fruit salad with yoghurt and nuts and seeds

DAY 5

BREAKFAST

Cornflakes with a chopped banana and a few nuts and seeds

LUNCH

Falafel with hoummos and salad on open rye bread sandwiches

DINNER

Cauliflower and broccoli cheese*

DESSERT

Tropical crumble*

DAY 6

BREAKFAST

Wake-up yoghurt shake*, plus 2 Ryvita with pure fruit spread

LUNCH

Rye bread sandwiches with fish, poultry, cheese or egg filling served with a salad

DINNER

Lamb kebabs* with assorted fresh vegetables and new potatoes

DESSERT

Banana with ice-cream or home-made vanilla custard

DAY 7

BREAKFAST

2 egg mushroom omelette with 100% pure rye bread

LUNCH

Home-made vegetable soup with oat cakes or Ryvita

DINNER

Pilchards in tomato sauce with salad and a jacket potato

DESSERT

Rye pancakes with fresh fruit or stewed fruit compôte or Yeo Valley fruit compôte, served with natural bio yoghurt or crème fraîche

Note: If you don't feel so well on oats, wait a few days before trying rye and replace the oats on days 4–7 with rice and corn products.

WEEK 7

If you have introduced both oats and rye successfully, without any symptoms or adverse effects, you can now move on to introducing foods containing white flour. If however, you have gained some weight or some of your old symptoms have returned to greet you, you should go back on to the basic diet, including dairy products, if you were fine with those, for another week or two until things settle down.

I have had many patients who have been so happy on Phase One of the Discovery Diet, and so pleased to be feeling good while at the same time losing weight, that they were reluctant to make any changes. So if you don't yet feel happy about appearing in public in the bikini of your choice, or simply felt better on the basic diet, feel free to continue with your current eating plan for as long as you like, for unlike most ordinary weight loss diets, it is an eating plan that is nutritionally balanced for the long-term.

Those of you who are going on to introduce foods containing white flour may be surprised to find that the introduction of white flour comes before wholemeal products, which are perceived to be better for us. While it may appear strange, sound reasoning is involved. Whole-grain products, including bran, have a much higher gluten content than refined white flour, and are therefore more likely to cause a reaction. So it is always advisable to start introducing foods made with white flour, like bread, pasta, pastry, pizza and sauces, to test the water.

The best thing to try first is French bread made with French flour, which is now widely available from most supermarkets in the UK, as French flour has far lower gluten content that British grown wheat. This means you can start tucking into baguettes, which you have probably been dreaming of for the last six weeks. Make sure you keep careful notes during this process and weigh yourself regularly, watching out for weight surges, flagging energy levels or bowel symptoms like bloating, wind or constipation or diarrhoea. You will see from this week's menu that we advise the introduction of small quantities of bread initially, gradually increasing the number of servings and portion sizes as the week progresses.

PHASE TWO – WEEK 7

WHITE FLOUR TRIAL
BREAKFAST
- Wake-up muesli* with chopped fresh fruit and semi-skimmed milk
- Scrambled eggs with a toasted bagel
- Bio yoghurt with chopped fresh fruit and Wake-up shake *
- 2 boiled eggs with white toasted soldiers
- Cornflakes with chopped unsalted nuts and seeds with semi-skimmed milk
- Porridge made with semi-skimmed milk with stewed apple, cinnamon and ginger
- Ryvita with nut butter and a banana
- Pancakes with stewed apple, sultanas and cinnamon and bio yoghurt
- 2 slices of white toast with pure fruit spread or a little honey

LUNCHES
- Baked beans on toast
- Hoummos and falafel with a mixed salad and pitta bread
- Spinach and mushroom quiche served with salad

- Oven roasted vegetables and hoummos served with ciabatta bread
- Tuna and pasta salad
- Cheese salad with French bread
- Tuna and mozzarella toasted sandwich
- Greek salad with pitta bread
- French bread pizza topped with tomatoes, basil, mozzarella, olives (and prawns)

DINNERS
- Fish in breadcrumbs with spinach, broccoli and new potatoes
- Grilled chicken breast marinated in lemon, garlic and black pepper with assorted fresh vegetables
- Flour tortillas with mince or beans, guacamole and salsa
- Spaghetti bolognaise
- Pasta with tomato and basil sauce with spinach, mushrooms and pine kernels
- Homemade pizza with topping of your choice
- Poached salmon with assorted fresh vegetables
- Mushroom quiche with a large salad and potato wedges
- Tomato and basil sauce with tagliatelle, sprinkled with a little grated parmesan cheese
- Cherry tomatoes, mozzarella and basil marinated in olive oil and balsamic vinegar served with fresh pasta

DESSERTS
- Apple charlotte*
- Pancakes* with stewed fruit of your choice or Yeo Valley fruit compôte and natural bio yoghurt or crème fraîche
- Apple pie and ice-cream or custard
- Summer berry crumble served with natural bio yoghurt
- Fresh fruit salad with toasted almonds and pumpkin seeds
- Summer pudding
- Bread and butter pudding with custard
- Stewed prunes and apricots served with natural yoghurt
- Banana custard with a few chopped nuts

SWEET SNACKS

- White muffin, toasted with pure fruit spread
- Cinnamon and raisin bagel
- Bread with honey
- White toast with sugar free jam
- Crackers and sugar free jam
- Crunchy oat cereal bar
- Bio fruit yoghurt
- Fresh fruit
- Cottage cheese, fresh pineapple and a few sunflower seeds
- Fruit smoothie

SAVOURY SNACKS

- Cheese on white toast
- Toast with nut butter or pure fruit jam
- Pitta bread with hoummos
- Rye bread with a little portion of cheese
- Oat cakes with nut butter or honey
- Small amounts of low fat cheese with toast or crackers
- Unsalted nuts and seeds
- Small piece of cheese and crackers with an apple
- Cheese and herb scone

WEEK 7 MENUS

DAY 1

BREAKFAST

Scrambled eggs with a piece of French bread

LUNCH

Jacket potato with baked beans

DINNER

Grilled chicken breast marinated in lemon, garlic and black pepper with assorted fresh vegetables

DESSERT

Apple charlotte*

WEEK 7 DIARY

DATE:

Please complete the diary on a daily basis and grade symptoms on a scale of 0-3

0 = NONE, 1 = MILD, 2 = MODERATE, 3 = SEVERE

Day 1

BREAKFAST . . . . LUNCH . . . .

DINNER . . . . SNACKS . . . .

EXERCISE . . . . SUPPLEMENTS . . . .

RELAXATION . . . . SYMPTOMS . . . .

REACTIONS . . . .

Day 2

BREAKFAST . . . . LUNCH . . . .

DINNER . . . . SNACKS . . . .

EXERCISE . . . . SUPPLEMENTS . . . .

RELAXATION . . . . SYMPTOMS . . . .

REACTIONS . . . .

Day 3

BREAKFAST . . . . LUNCH . . . .

DINNER . . . . SNACKS . . . .

EXERCISE . . . . SUPPLEMENTS . . . .

RELAXATION . . . . SYMPTOMS . . . .

REACTIONS . . . .

Day 4

BREAKFAST . . . . LUNCH . . . .

DINNER . . . . SNACKS . . . .

EXERCISE . . . . SUPPLEMENTS . . . .

RELAXATION . . . . SYMPTOMS . . . .

REACTIONS . . . .

Day 5

BREAKFAST . . . . LUNCH . . . .

DINNER . . . . SNACKS . . . .

EXERCISE . . . . SUPPLEMENTS . . . .

RELAXATION . . . . SYMPTOMS . . . .

REACTIONS . . . .

Day 6

BREAKFAST . . . . LUNCH . . . .

DINNER . . . . SNACKS . . . .

EXERCISE . . . . SUPPLEMENTS . . . .

RELAXATION . . . . SYMPTOMS . . . .

REACTIONS . . . .

Day 7

BREAKFAST . . . . LUNCH . . . .

DINNER . . . . SNACKS . . . .

EXERCISE . . . . SUPPLEMENTS . . . .

RELAXATION . . . . SYMPTOMS . . . .

REACTIONS . . . .

DAY 2

BREAKFAST
Bio yoghurt with chopped fresh fruit and Wake-up shake *

LUNCH
Tuna and mozzarella toasted sandwich

DINNER
Pasta with tomato and basil sauce with spinach, mushrooms and pine kernels

DESSERT
Summer berry crumble served with natural bio yoghurt

DAY 3

BREAKFAST
2 boiled eggs with white toasted soldiers

LUNCH
Spinach and mushroom quiche served with salad

DINNER
Homemade pizza with topping of your choice

DESSERT
Fresh fruit salad with toasted almonds and pumpkin seeds

DAY 4

BREAKFAST
Pancakes with stewed apple, sultanas and cinnamon and bio yoghurt

LUNCH
Hoummos and falafel with a mixed salad

DINNER
Poached salmon with assorted fresh vegetables

DESSERT
Bread and butter pudding with custard

DAY 5

BREAKFAST
Wake-up muesli* with chopped fresh fruit and semi-skimmed milk

LUNCH

Sandwich with cottage cheese, sweetcorn and a large salad

DINNER

Spaghetti bolognaise or tomato and basil sauce with tagliatelle, sprinkled with a little grated parmesan cheese

DESSERT

Stewed prunes and apricots served with natural yoghurt

DAY 6

BREAKFAST

Toasted bagel with nut butter and a mashed banana

LUNCH

Oven roasted vegetables and hommos served with ciabatta bread

DINNER

Jacket potato with tinned mackerel in tomato sauce, served with a large salad

DESSERT

Apple pie with custard

DAY 7

BREAKFAST

Cornflakes with chopped unsalted nuts and seeds with semi-skimmed milk

LUNCH

Greek salad with pitta bread

DINNER

Pasta with tomato and basil sauce with spinach, mushrooms and pine kernels

DESSERT

Summer pudding home-made custard or natural yoghurt

Note: If you don't feel so well on white flour, wait a few days before trying the wholemeal trial.

WEEK 8

If weight loss has been your main motivation for following the Discovery Diet, be wary about introducing wholewheat before you have reached your target weight. In my experience, many people who are not in brilliant nutritional shape, and whose immune system may not be operating in an optimum fashion, may retain fluid as part of an adverse chemical reaction to the wholewheat or bran. It is therefore advisable to leave the re-introduction of wholewheat or wheat bran until you have achieved your target weight, and have overcome any bowel symptoms or fatigue, if they were part of your 'baggage'.

Once you are feeling well and have lost the desired weight, feel free to reintroduce wholewheat products gradually over a period of a week or two, while keeping careful notes of any symptoms that may occur and watching your weight like a hawk. If the scales show that the pounds are creeping back on – beware. It may be that at this point you can tolerate wholewheat in small quantities, which will mean that you can eat it 'socially' rather than as part of your everyday diet.

If the reaction to wholewheat is severe, it is best to exclude it completely from your diet for at least the next few months, before having another attempt at its re-introduction. You will have discovered by now that there are plenty of delicious alternatives freely available, and it may even be that you are quite happy with your current diet, and have stopped pining for wholewheat some time ago.

If you decide that wheat, or wholewheat, are no go areas at the moment, you simply need to go back on to the basic diet for the next week or two in order to drop the pounds you gained while doing the experiment. You may be surprised by the rapid loss of weight once off wheat again, but remember that fluid may have collected to dilute the chemical reaction in your body which, once off wheat, is now no longer required.

Compared with how you felt when you started the plan, by now you should be feeling fabulous. As you progress through the last week of the plan, give yourself a gold star, but make a point of not getting complacent. Consider the dietary and lifestyle changes you have had to make to get to this point, and think twice before returning to your old habits.

By the end of this week you will essentially have completed your voyage of discovery on the Discovery Diet, so we can then move on to put the longer-term plan together.

PHASE TWO – WEEK 8

WHOLEMEAL FLOUR TRIAL

BREAKFAST

- Wholemeal toast with nut butter or pure fruit spread
- Scrambled eggs on wholemeal toast
- Shredded wheat with chopped pecan nuts, fresh pear and semi-skimmed milk
- Wholewheat muesli with semi-skimmed milk or bio yoghurt
- Natural bio yoghurt with Wake-up shake*
- Stewed prunes with natural bio yoghurt and crunchy oat cereal
- Pancakes made with wholemeal flour, served with stewed apple, sultanas and cinnamon
- Wholemeal muffin with a poached egg, and mushrooms and tomatoes lightly sautéed in olive oil

LUNCHES

- Pilchards in tomato sauce with salad and wholemeal bread
- Falafel with hoummos and a large salad in a wholemeal pitta bread
- Scrambled eggs and baked beans on wholemeal toast

- Chicken, avocado and tomato wholemeal sandwich
- Omelette with a large salad
- Wholemeal mushroom quiche with salad
- Cherry tomato, basil and mozzarella salad with wholemeal pitta bread
- Homemade vegetable soup with a chunk of wholemeal bread

DINNERS
- Grilled plaice with fresh vegetables and brown rice
- Turkey and green pepper kebabs with hoummos, salad and wholemeal pitta bread
- Stir-fry vegetables (and chicken) with brown rice or egg noodles
- Wholewheat spinach and goats' cheese pizza with salad
- Poached salmon with assorted fresh vegetables
- Ratatouille with wholemeal pasta and a salad with olive oil and balsamic vinegar
- Oven-roasted Mediterranean vegetables with mozzarella cheese
- Wholemeal salmon and broccoli quiche with salad
- Wholemeal pasta with a tomato and herb sauce
- Cold chicken with a jacket potato and large salad

DESSERTS
- Wholemeal apple and cinnamon crumble with homemade custard or ice-cream
- Wholemeal pancakes with stewed summer berries and Greek yoghurt
- Fresh fruit salad with yoghurt and a few nuts and seeds
- Wholemeal date slice with natural bio yoghurt
- Natural bio yoghurt with honey and a banana
- Wholemeal bread and butter pudding with homemade custard
- Grilled pineapple marinated in lemon juice, and a little brown sugar, served with toasted pecans and fromage frais

SWEET SNACKS
- Wholemeal muffin, toasted with pure fruit spread
- Wholemeal fruit scone
- Granary bread with honey
- Crunchy cereal bar
- Bio fruit yoghurt
- Fresh fruit
- Fruit smoothie

SAVOURY SNACKS
- Cheese on wholemeal toast
- Wholemeal toast with nut butter or sugar-free jam
- Wholemeal pitta bread with hoummos
- Rye bread with a little portion of cheese
- Oat cakes with nut butter or honey
- Small amounts of low fat cheese with rice cakes or alternative toast
- Unsalted nuts and seeds
- Small piece of cheese and wholemeal crackers with an apple
- Wholemeal cheese and herb scone

WEEK 8 MENUS

DAY 1
BREAKFAST
Wholemeal toast with nut butter or pure fruit spread
LUNCH
Jacket potato with hoummos and a large salad
DINNER
Grilled plaice with fresh vegetables and brown rice
DESSERT
Wholemeal bread and butter pudding with ice-cream or homemade custard

WEEK 8 DIARY

DATE:

Please complete the diary on a daily basis and grade symptoms on a scale of 0-3

0 = NONE, 1 = MILD, 2 = MODERATE, 3 = SEVERE

Day 1

BREAKFAST . . . . LUNCH . . . .

DINNER . . . . SNACKS . . . .

EXERCISE . . . . SUPPLEMENTS . . . .

RELAXATION . . . . SYMPTOMS . . . .

REACTIONS . . . .

Day 2

BREAKFAST . . . . LUNCH . . . .

DINNER . . . . SNACKS . . . .

EXERCISE . . . . SUPPLEMENTS . . . .

RELAXATION . . . . SYMPTOMS . . . .

REACTIONS . . . .

Day 3

BREAKFAST . . . . LUNCH . . . .

DINNER . . . . SNACKS . . . .

EXERCISE . . . . SUPPLEMENTS . . . .

RELAXATION . . . . SYMPTOMS . . . .

REACTIONS . . . .

Day 4

BREAKFAST . . . . LUNCH . . . .

DINNER . . . . SNACKS . . . .

EXERCISE . . . . SUPPLEMENTS . . . .

RELAXATION . . . . SYMPTOMS . . . .

REACTIONS . . . .

Day 5

BREAKFAST . . . . LUNCH . . . .

DINNER . . . . SNACKS . . . .

EXERCISE . . . . SUPPLEMENTS . . . .

RELAXATION . . . . SYMPTOMS . . . .

REACTIONS . . . .

Day 6

BREAKFAST . . . . LUNCH . . . .

DINNER . . . . SNACKS . . . .

EXERCISE . . . . SUPPLEMENTS . . . .

RELAXATION . . . . SYMPTOMS . . . .

REACTIONS . . . .

Day 7

BREAKFAST . . . . LUNCH . . . .

DINNER . . . . SNACKS . . . .

EXERCISE . . . . SUPPLEMENTS . . . .

RELAXATION . . . . SYMPTOMS . . . .

REACTIONS . . . .

DAY 2

BREAKFAST
Wake-up muesli* with semi-skimmed milk and natural bio yoghurt

LUNCH
Wholemeal mushroom quiche with salad

DINNER
Stir-fry vegetables (and chicken) with brown rice or egg noodles

DESSERT
Grilled pineapple marinated in lemon juice, and sugar, served with toasted pecans and Greek yoghurt

DAY 3

BREAKFAST
Wholemeal muffin with a poached egg, and mushrooms and tomatoes lightly sautéed in olive oil

LUNCH
Homemade vegetable soup with a chunk of wholemeal bread

DINNER
Grilled salmon brushed with pesto with assorted fresh vegetables

DESSERT
Natural yoghurt with honey and a banana

DAY 4

BREAKFAST
Pancakes made with wholemeal flour, served with stewed apple, sultanas and cinnamon

LUNCH
Oven-roasted Mediterranean vegetables with mozzarella cheese

DINNER
Turkey and apricot kebabs with hoummos, salad and wholemeal pitta bread

DESSERT
Wholemeal date slice with natural yoghurt

DAY 5

BREAKFAST

Wholewheat muesli with semi-skimmed milk or yoghurt

LUNCH

Chicken, avocado and tomato wholemeal sandwich

DINNER

Wholemeal salmon and broccoli quiche with salad

DESSERT

Fresh fruit salad with yoghurt and a few nuts and seeds

DAY 6

BREAKFAST

Shredded Wheat with chopped pecan nuts, fresh pear with
milk or soya milk

LUNCH

Mushroom omelette with a large salad

DINNER

Wholewheat spinach and goats' cheese pizza with salad

DESSERT

Wholemeal pancakes with stewed summer berries and Greek
yoghurt

DAY 7

BREAKFAST

Scrambled eggs on wholemeal toast

LUNCH

Jacket potato with pilchards in tomato sauce and a large
salad

DINNER

Ratatouille with wholemeal pasta and a salad with olive oil,
lemon juice and balsamic vinegar

DESSERT

Wholemeal apple and cinnamon crumble with homemade
custard or natural yoghurt

The Discovery Diet – Grand Review

By the time you reach the final section of the Discovery Diet you should be looking good, feeling well and proud of your achievement. The general consensus is that the voyage through this plan is a learning curve through previously untrodden territory. You now know how to interpret your body's messages and have become familiar with what it likes and dislikes.

Formulating your long-term plan

You will probably be only too aware of any reactions experienced during the two phases of the Discovery Diet, but it is still worth setting a little time aside both to review your progress and to make a plan for the future.

- As you look through the weekly charts make a list of any foods or drinks that definitely seemed to cause a reaction, which will be known as your 'black list'. Make another list of items that you are currently unsure of, your 'grey list'.

- You will need to concentrate on all the products on your 'white list' (the foods and drinks you seemed to thrive on) for the next few weeks, taking care to omit items from both the grey and black lists from your diet.

- When you feel the time is right, for example when you are feeling really well, or when you have reached and maintained your target weight for a few months, re-test the grey list by introducing them back into your diet one by one, as before leaving five days between foods.

- Another few months down the line, re-test the remaining foods on the grey list gradually, one by one as before. Sometimes when the body is in better nutritional shape the tolerance to certain foods and drinks improves.

- The foods and drinks that remain on both the grey list and the black list may be tested again several months down the line, but always individually, leaving plenty of time for any reaction to rear its head.

Review

White list = Foods and drinks on which you seem well
Grey list = Foods and drinks of which you are currently unsure
Black list = Foods and drinks to which you had a reaction

	White List	Grey List	Black List
Phase I			

Phase II			

Phase III			

Remember the most important factor is that you continue to feel well and in good communication with your body. Once you get to know what your body likes and dislikes you may even decide to blow caution to the wind on certain social occasions, knowing that you may pay for it later. At least now you are armed with the knowledge of how best to feed your body and keep it happy.

The Discovery Diet in the long-term

To continue losing weight

If you had a considerable amount of weight to lose, and have not achieved your target weight by the end of the Discovery Diet, there is nothing to stop you continuing for as many months as you wish. Unlike other weight-loss diets you have followed this diet is designed to be followed in the long-term. You will have gathered by now that it provides you with all the important nutrients your body needs in order to thrive.

Once you have completed your weight-loss programme

There is no need to revert to your old way of eating when you have completed the Discovery Diet. It will be much better for your health and well-being in the long-term if you remain on the regime, perhaps increasing the portion sizes a little, or adding in some of the little treats listed in the dessert section, for example. There is no harm in deviating from your basic diet on special occasions or at holiday times, as you are now armed with the knowledge of what your body really needs on a regular basis. And, I firmly believe that when you are well, 'a little of what you fancy does you good'.

Supplements for the long-term

While at the WNAS we are not recommending long-term pill popping across the board, there are times when supplements will improve the quality of life, especially when taken in reduced doses over a period of time. The supplements that may be required during the various phases of life will vary.

During the Discovery Diet you will have had the opportunity to experiment with supplements that you felt were indicated. As we are all so different, your long-term supplement programme, should you decide that supplements are necessary, will be the result of trial and error over the months, until you find the regime that seems to suit you. There will be times when you need to change your regime, for example when you are actively planning to conceive, are pregnant or breastfeeding.

Further suggested reading is our book *The Natural Health Bible*, which outlines over 120 different conditions, with full details about both what your doctor has to offer and what you can do to self-help. See page 335 for details.

Keep fit and make time for yourself

Unfortunately, most of us have to work at remaining in good physical and mental shape. While it may take a while and some in-depth personal persuasion to get a regular exercise programme established, I think you will agree that it gives you a regular infusion of that 'feel-good-factor'. So don't get complacent at the end of the Discovery Diet and think you feel so well there is no need to continue. Many have made that mistake before and lived to regret it! Enjoy your exercise time, and make time to relax on a regular basis, even if it's only for 15 minutes per day.

Making time for yourself is probably one of the most important long-term resolutions you should be considering. Somehow when we are feeling good we forget how important healthy eating, exercise and relaxation are. If you lead a hectic life I suggest you write your exercise and relaxation time into your diary like any business or a hairdressing appointment. That way you stand a good chance of preserving that special time for yourself.

We all need time to reflect on our lives, on decisions that need to be made, or indeed on our achievements. The time you invest in exercise and relaxation will be repaid to you in terms of increased energy and elevated mood. When you feel positive, happy and energetic you are bound to achieve more in life, and to attract more interesting company.

Having helped tens of thousands of individuals to help themselves to better health, I really believe that in the final analysis it is up to each of us to invest in ourselves. Once armed with the knowledge, which of course you now are, the quality of your health in the long-term is very much in your own hands. You may regard this as a somewhat daunting prospect, but it very definitely puts you in the driving seat, and the only side-effects that you are likely to experience are that you will be looking good and feeling fine for a long time to come.

CHAPTER **23**

The Discovery Diet Recipes

BREAKFAST – PHASE ONE

WAKE-UP MUESLI
Makes 10–12 servings

$2^{1}/_{2}$ mugs puffed rice
2 mugs Cornflakes
$^{1}/_{2}$ mug sunflower seeds
$^{1}/_{2}$ mug chopped almonds
$^{2}/_{3}$ mug organic raisins

1. Mix the ingredients together and store in a sealed container.
2. Serve with chopped fresh fruit and the appropriate yoghurt or milk of your phase.

Note If you are constipated you will need to sprinkle 1–2 tablespoons of organic linseeds on to your muesli each morning for the best results.

WAKE-UP SPRINKLE
Makes 18 tablespoons (1 level tablespoon = 1 serving)

Three servings per week are allowed until you have reached
your target weight. Use organic seeds where possible.

½ mug almonds
½ mug sunflower seeds
⅓ mug pumpkin seeds
¼ mug golden linseeds

1. Grind the ingredients together in a blender to a coarse
   powder consistency.
2. Store in a sealed container. This gives a new dimension to
   breakfasts, salads and desserts.

WAKE-UP YOGHURT SHAKE
Makes 2 large servings

1 large carton of soya yoghurt
3 portions fruit of your choice, skinned and cut into segments
ice cubes (optional)

1. Blend the ingredients together in a liquidiser and serve
   immediately.
Variation Blend in 2 tablespoons Wake-up sprinkle*

MIXED BERRY BONANZA
Serves 2

1 cup frozen mixed berries (partially thawed)
1 banana
450ml (¾ pint) soya milk
1 cup natural bio soya yoghurt
1 tbsp ground almonds

1. Blend the fruit with the soya milk and yoghurt.
2. Stir in the ground almonds thoroughly and serve immediately.

PANCAKES
Serves 4

125g (4oz) Dove's Farm gluten-free flour
1 small egg
300ml (½ pint) soya milk
a little oil

1. Make a thin batter with the flour, egg and milk.
2. Use kitchen paper to wipe a small non-stick frying pan with a little oil and heat until the oil is smoking.
3. Pour a generous 2 tablespoons of batter into the pan and swirl it around to cover the base. Cook for 60 seconds.
4. Flip it over and cook for a further few seconds. Set aside.
5. Repeat the procedure until you have used up all the batter.

GLUTEN-FREE MUESLI
Makes 10–12 servings

2 mugs brown rice flakes
1 mug buckwheat flakes
½ mug sunflower seeds
½ mug chopped almonds
½ mug pumpkin seeds
⅔ mug organic raisins (optional)

1. Mix the ingredients together and store in a sealed container.
2. Serve with chopped fresh fruit and the appropriate yoghurt or milk of your phase.

MUSHROOM AND TOMATO OMELETTE
Serves 1

2 medium eggs
soya milk
50g (2oz) mushrooms
2 ripe tomatoes
olive oil
freshly ground black pepper

1. Crack the eggs and beat together with a little soya milk. Season with black pepper and little salt. Put to one side.
2. Lightly sauté the mushrooms and tomatoes in a large frying pan in olive oil until golden.
3. Pour the egg and milk mixture over the mushrooms and tomatoes into the frying pan and cook for 2–3 minutes until the underside is golden and the top is bubbling.
4. Either turn the omelette in the pan to cook the top, or put under a medium hot grill until the eggs are cooked and the omelette is firm.
5. Serve with baked beans for an extra special breakfast.

BREAKFAST PHASE TWO

WAKE-UP YOGHURT SHAKE
Makes 2 large servings

1 large carton of natural bio yoghurt or Yeo Valley apricot
  flavour
3 portions fruit of your choice, skinned and cut into segments
ice cubes (optional)

1. Blend the ingredients together in a liquidiser and serve immediately.

SWISS MUESLI
Serves 2

2 cups porridge oats
1 apple, peeled and grated
1 cup raisins
300ml (½ pint) pint apple juice or soya milk
1 tbsp chopped almonds
1 cup natural bio yoghurt
sprinkling of ground cinnamon and ginger

1. Soak the porridge oats, grated apple and raisins for at least half an hour in the apple juice or soya milk.
2. Stir in the chopped almonds and yoghurt and serve with a sprinkling of ground cinnamon and ginger.

RYE AND RICE PANCAKES
Serves 4

50g (2oz) rye flour
50g (2oz) brown rice flour
1 small egg
300ml (½ pint) soya milk or semi-skimmed milk
a little oil

1. Make a thin batter with the rye and rice flour, egg and milk.
2. Use kitchen paper to wipe a small non-stick frying pan with a little oil and heat until the oil is smoking.
3. Pour a generous 2 tablespoons of batter into the pan and swirl it around to cover the base. Cook for 60 seconds.
4. Flip the pancake over and cook for a further few seconds. Set aside.
5. Repeat the procedure until you have used up all the batter.

PANCAKES
Serves 4

125g (4oz) white plain flour
1 small egg
300ml (½ pint) soya milk or semi-skimmed milk
a little oil

1. Make a thin batter with the flour, egg and milk.
2. Use kitchen paper to wipe a small non-stick frying pan with a little oil and heat until the oil is smoking.
3. Pour a generous 2 tablespoons of batter into the pan and swirl it around to cover the base. Cook for 60 seconds.
4. Flip the pancake over and cook for a further few seconds. Set aside.
5. Repeat the procedure until you have used up all the batter.

SOUPS – PHASE ONE AND TWO

CHICKEN AND SPINACH SOUP
Serves 4

2 chicken breasts, skinned and each chopped into 8 pieces
600ml (1 pint) water
10ml (2 tsp) sunflower oil
1 onion, finely chopped
150g (5oz) spinach, stalks removed and leaves shredded
600ml (1 pint) soya milk

1. Place the chicken and water in a saucepan, bring to the boil and simmer for 45 minutes.
2. Heat the oil and gently fry the onions for 2 minutes until translucent.
3. Remove the onions with a slotted spoon and add to the chicken and liquid.

4. Add the spinach, season with black pepper to taste, and cook for a further 5 minutes.
5. Add the soya milk and heat through before serving.

SWEET POTATO, BROCCOLI AND SPINACH SOUP
Serves 6–8

10ml (2 tsp) sunflower oil
1 onion, finely chopped
1 large sweet potato, peeled and diced
450ml (¾ pint) vegetable stock
1 large head of broccoli
225g (8oz) spinach
150ml (¼ pint) soya milk
seasoning to taste

1. Heat the oil in a large saucepan and soften the onion without browning.
2. Add the sweet potato and coat in the juices.
3. Add the vegetable stock, bring to the boil and simmer until the sweet potato starts to soften.
4. Finally, add the broccoli and spinach and continue cooking over a gentle heat until all the vegetables are cooked through.
5. Blend the ingredients in the pan with a hand blender or pour into a liquidiser. Blend until smooth.
6. Stir in the soya milk and season to taste. A little more soya milk can be added for a thinner consistency.

PUY LENTIL SOUP
Serves 6–8

450g (1lb) puy lentils
1 litre (1¾ pints) water
2 tbsp sunflower oil
1 large onion, peeled and finely chopped

2 garlic cloves, crushed
1.4 litres (2½ pints) vegetable stock
2 sticks celery, trimmed and chopped
1 large carrot, peeled and chopped
1 bay leaf
freshly ground black pepper

1. Place the puy lentils and water in a pan and bring to the boil. Boil for 2 minutes, then remove from the heat and leave to stand for 2 hours, covered. Drain.
2. Heat the oil in a saucepan and lightly brown the onion. Add the garlic and mix well.
3. Stir in the drained lentils, add the stock and bring to the boil.
4. Add the celery, carrots, bay leaf and black pepper.
5. Simmer for 45–60 minutes until the lentils are tender, then remove the bay leaf.
6. Half, or all the soup can be puréed in a blender or food processor.

LUNCHES – PHASE ONE AND TWO

SEAFOOD SALAD
Serves 6

350g (12oz) cod fillet
½ white cabbage, trimmed
225g (8oz) peeled prawns
125g (4oz) cooked mussels, shelled
1 onion, grated
125g (4oz) carrots, grated
½ teaspoon chopped fresh dill
olive oil dressing, shop bought or homemade

1. Steam the cod until tender, then remove the skin and

flake the fish. Leave to cool.
2. Shred the cabbage finely, then rinse and drain well. Pat dry with a clean cloth or kitchen paper.
3. Mix the cod, cabbage, prawns, mussels, onions, carrots and dill together.
4. Toss the salad in the olive oil dressing.

PEPPER AND LENTIL SALAD
Serves 4

1 large red pepper, de-seeded and chopped
1 large green pepper, de-seeded and chopped
1 onion, finely chopped
10 pitted black olives, halved
1 tbsp chopped fresh thyme
50g (2oz) Puy lentils, cooked
4 tbsp olive oil
4 tbsp lemon juice
1 garlic clove, crushed
black pepper to taste

1. In a large bowl, mix together the red pepper, green pepper, onion, olives, thyme and lentils.
2. Whisk the oil, lemon, garlic and black pepper together and pour on to the lentil mixture. Mix well to coat all the ingredients.

SALAD NIÇOISE
Serves 4

4 medium potatoes, scrubbed
4 medium tomatoes, cut into wedges
200g (7oz) can tuna in olive oil, drained and flaked
1 small crisp lettuce, separated into leaves
black pepper to taste
3 hard boiled eggs, shelled and cut into wedges

50g (2oz) can anchovies in oil, drained
10 black olives
olive oil dressing, homemade or shop bought

1. Cook the potatoes in boiling salted water for 15–20 minutes or until tender. Drain, cool, then cut into bite-sized pieces.
2. Mix the potato, tomatoes and tuna together.
3. Arrange the lettuce on a serving platter and spoon the tuna mixture into the middle. Sprinkle with black pepper.
4. Arrange the egg, anchovies and olives on top of the salad and pour over the olive oil dressing.

HERB TOFU
Serves 4

10ml (2 tsp) vegetable oil
1 small red pepper, seeded and thinly sliced
1 clove of garlic, crushed
170g (6oz) tofu, cubed
½ tablespoon of chopped parsley

1. Heat the oil in a frying pan.
2. Add the red pepper and garlic and fry for 2–3 minutes.
3. Add the tofu and parsley and continue to stir-fry until the tofu is heated through. Serve immediately.

TUNA JACKETS
Serves 4

15ml (1 tbsp) sunflower oil
1 red, 1 yellow and 1 green pepper, cored, seeded and diced
60ml (4 tbsp) white wine vinegar
30ml (2 tbsp) wholegrain mustard
200g (7oz) can tuna in oil, drained and flaked
125g (4oz) can sweetcorn, drained

4 hot baked potatoes
freshly ground black pepper

1. Heat the oil, add the diced peppers and sauté for 5 minutes. Add the vinegar and mustard and cook for 5 minutes, stirring.
2. Stir in the flaked tuna and sweetcorn.
3. Cut the tops off the potatoes and scoop out the centres. Chop the potato and stir it into half the pepper relish mixture. Season with black pepper to taste.
4. Spoon the potato mixture back into the potato jackets. Serve the remaining relish separately.

SPINACH AND AVOCADO SALAD
Serves 4

1 bag of baby spinach leaves
200g (7oz) avocado, sliced
12 black olives, stoned and quartered

Dressing
10ml (2tsp) olive oil
15ml (1tbsp) lemon juice (fresh)
1 garlic clove, crushed

1. Combine the spinach, avocado and olives in a bowl.
2. Mix the oil, lemon juice and garlic together and pour this dressing over the salad.
3. Lightly toss the salad until it is coated with the dressing and serve.
4. Ideal served as an accompaniment to chicken and fish.

CHICKPEA DIPS WITH CRUDITÉ
Serves 8

2 x 350g (15oz) cans chickpeas, drained and rinsed

1 garlic clove, crushed
15ml (1tbsp) lemon juice (fresh)
25ml (1floz) olive oil
175ml (6floz) natural soya yoghurt
freshly ground black pepper
4 teaspoons freshly chopped parsley
10ml (2tsp) tomato purée
sprigs of parsley and strips of red pepper and pieces of sliced
    lemon to garnish
selection of raw vegetables (peppers, radishes, carrots, celery,
    cucumber) to serve.

1. Place the chickpeas in a blender or food processor and
   blend until smooth.
2. Add the garlic, lemon juice, olive oil and soya yoghurt
   and mix well. Add the pepper to taste.
3. Transfer one-third of the mixture to a small serving bowl.
   Divide the rest between 2 small mixing bowls.
4. Add the chopped parsley to one, stir well and transfer to a
   small serving bowl.
5. Add the tomato purée to the other, stir well and transfer
   to a small serving bowl. Adjust seasoning if necessary.
6. Garnish the herb dip with sprigs of parsley, the tomato
   dip with red pepper and the plain dip with the pieces of
   lemon.
7. Chop the vegetables into sticks. Arrange on a serving dish
   around the dips.

DINNER – PHASE ONE

LAMB KEBABS
Serves 4

Marinade
3 tbsp soya yoghurt
juice ½ lime

2 garlic cloves, crushed
3 tbsp chopped fresh coriander
1 tbsp chopped fresh mint
1 tsp each curry powder and cumin
pinch each of salt and cayenne pepper

450g (1lb) lamb neck fillet, trimmed and cut into chunks
1 green pepper
1 red pepper
1 large onion
450g (1lb) button mushrooms

1. Combine the marinade ingredients in a large bowl. Add the lamb and stir. Cover and chill for at least 2 hours.
2. Thread the lamb, peppers, onions and mushrooms on to skewers in an alternate pattern. Cook for 4–6 minutes on each side (either on a barbecue on under a hot grill). Serve with lime wedges.

CUMIN CHICKEN
Serves 2

1 tsp vegetable oil
1 tsp cumin seeds
2 x 125g (4oz) chicken breast fillets, cubed
½ red pepper, chopped
3 spring onions, chopped
1 tsp finely chopped root ginger
300ml (½ pint) of stock
cornflour
water

1. Heat oil in saucepan, add the cumin seeds and stir until they start popping.
2. Add chicken, pepper, onions and ginger; stir for 3 minutes.

3. Add the stock, bring to the boil, simmer for 5 minutes.
4. Add the cornflour (mixed into paste with water), and simmer for a further 5 minutes before serving.

FISH STEW WITH PEPPERS
Serves 4

30ml (2 tbsp) sunflower oil
450g (1lb) canned peeled tomatoes
1 red chilli, seeded and finely chopped
2 green peppers, cored, seeded and sliced
2 medium onions, finely chopped
3 garlic cloves, crushed
50ml (2 floz) dry white wine (avoid on a yeast-free diet)
1 tsp dried thyme
1 bay leaf
900g (2lb) sole fillets, cut into 2.5cm (1 inch) cubes
450g (1lb) small new potatoes, scrubbed, cooked until just tender and kept warm

1. In an ovenproof dish heat the oil and add the tomatoes, including the juice, and the chilli. Stirring occasionally, cook for 15 minutes or until the mixture is thick.
2. Stir in the green peppers, onions, garlic, wine, thyme, bay leaf and fish cubes. Cover the dish, reduce the heat to low, and cook for 10 minutes, stirring occasionally.
3. Add the potatoes and turn them over in the fish mixture. Cover again and cook for a further 5 minutes, until the fish flakes easily when tested with a fork.
4. Discard the bay leaf and serve at once.

PRAWN AND VEGETABLE STIR-FRY
Serves 4

3 tbsp (45ml) vegetable oil
125g (4oz) broccoli, divided into florets

125g (4oz) carrots, cut into small matchstick-size pieces
125g (4oz) leeks, thinly sliced
225g (8oz) peeled prawns
55g (2oz) courgettes, thinly sliced
125g (4oz) Chinese leaves, roughly chopped
1 apple, cored and diced
1 tbsp grated ginger
125g (4oz) onions, chopped
1 tbsp (15ml) lemon juice

1. Heat oil in a wok or large frying pan, add the broccoli, carrots and leeks and cook for 3 minutes.
2. Add the prawns, courgettes, Chinese leaves, apple, ginger, onions and lemon juice.
3. Stir-fry for a further 2 minutes.
4. Serve immediately.

SALMON STEAKS WITH GINGER
Serves 2

2 salmon steaks
30ml (2 tbsp) lemon juice
2.5cm (1 inch) square of fresh ginger, peeled and finely chopped
freshly ground black pepper to taste

1. Place each salmon steak on a large piece of foil. Add 1 tablespoon of lemon juice and half the chopped ginger to each steak. Season with a little black pepper.
2. Wrap the steaks individually in foil to make two parcels and bake in a preheated oven at 180°C/350°F/Gas 4 for 20 minutes. Serve hot with vegetable or cold with a salad.

CHICKEN WITH ALMONDS
Serves 4

4 chicken breasts
15g (½ oz) butter or margarine
150ml (¼ pint) water
a few black peppercorns
75g (3oz) flaked almonds

1. Skin the chicken and brush with melted butter or margarine.
2. Place water and peppercorns in an ovenprooof dish. Place the chicken in the water and cover with foil. Bake for 15 minutes in the a preheated oven at 180°C/350°F/Gas 4.
3. Remove the foil and sprinkle with flaked almonds. Return to the oven for a further 15 minutes, or until the chicken is tender and the almonds have browned.
4. Serve with steamed vegetables, e.g. new potatoes and broccoli.

TURKEY AND CHICKPEAS WITH RICE
Serves 4

50g (2oz) margarine
12 pickling onions
900g (2lb) turkey breast, cut into 2.5cm (1 inch) cubes
125g (4oz) chickpeas, soaked overnight and drained
225ml (8floz) vegetable stock
freshly ground black pepper
1 tsp cumin seeds
pinch of turmeric
450g (1lb) long grain rice, washed, soaked in cold water for 30 minutes and drained

1. Melt the margarine in a large pan over a moderate heat. Add the onions and turkey cubes and cook, stirring and turning, for 5–8 minutes, until the onions are golden.

2. Add the chickpeas, stock and enough water to cover the mixture completely.
3. Add the pepper to taste, cumin and turmeric to the pan and stir well to blend. Cover the pan and cook for 1¼ hours or until the turkey and chickpeas are tender.
4. Raise the heat and bring the liquid to the boil. Stir in the rice. Cover the pan, reduce the heat and simmer for 15–20 minutes or until the rice is tender and the liquid absorbed.
5. Remove the pan from the heat, spoon the mixture into a warmed serving dish and serve immediately.

SPANISH RICE
Serves 3–4

3 tbsp olive oil
2 onions, thinly sliced
2 garlic cloves, crushed
1 green pepper, cored, seeded and thinly sliced
2 red peppers, cored, seeded and thinly sliced
350g (12oz) mushrooms, thinly sliced
1 x 400g (14oz) can chopped tomatoes
40g (1½oz) stoned green olives (optional)
1 tsp dried oregano
½ tsp basil
freshly ground black pepper
150g (5oz) cooked brown rice

1. Heat the oil in a large frying pan. Add the onions and garlic and cook for 5–7 minutes, stirring occasionally.
2. Add the green and red peppers and cook for 4 minutes, stirring frequently. Add the mushrooms, tomatoes, with their juices, olives (if using), oregano, basil and pepper and cook, stirring occasionally for 3 minutes.
3. Add the rice to the pan and cook for 3–4 minutes, stirring constantly until the rice is heated through, and serve immediately.

STUFFED PEPPERS
Serves 2

2 medium red peppers
olive oil
1 red onion, finely chopped
125g (4oz) carrot, grated
2 small courgettes, grated
75g (3oz) button mushrooms, chopped
1 clove garlic, crushed
freshly ground black pepper
handful chopped fresh parsley
125g (4oz) cooked brown rice
75g (3oz) cooked kidney beans
125g (4oz) canned sweetcorn
75g (3oz) baby plum tomatoes

1. Halve the peppers lengthways, scoop out the seeds and
   steam for 10 minutes.
2. Heat the olive oil in a frying pan and sauté the onion,
   carrot, courgette, mushrooms and garlic until softened.
   Season with black pepper and add the fresh parsley.
3. Combine the sautéed ingredients with the brown rice,
   kidney beans, sweetcorn and tomatoes and pile into the
   peppers.
4. Place peppers in an ovenproof dish, cover and cook for 15
   minutes at 200°C/400°F/Gas 6 until cooked and golden.
   Serve with a large mixed salad.

MUSHROOM AND HERB RISOTTO
Serves 4

2 tbsp olive oil
1 medium onion, finely chopped
1 clove garlic, crushed
1 red pepper, seeded and sliced

1 green pepper, seeded and sliced
125g (4oz) courgettes, thinly sliced
225g (8oz) chestnut mushrooms, washed and sliced
225g (8oz) brown rice
300ml (½ pint) chicken or vegetable stock
150ml (¼ pint) white wine
1 tbsp fresh parsley, chopped
1 tbsp fresh basil, torn
freshly ground black pepper

1. Heat the olive oil in a large saucepan, and sauté the onion, garlic, peppers, courgettes and mushrooms until softened.
2. Add the rice to the pan, mixing until all grains are thoroughly coated in the oil. Stir for about 2 minutes.
3. Pour the hot stock and wine into the saucepan and bring to the boil.
4. Reduce the heat and simmer with the lid off for 15–20 minutes until the rice has absorbed the liquid. Add the herbs and season with freshly ground black pepper.

DINNER – PHASE TWO

FRITTATA

125g (4oz) small new potatoes
125g (4oz) shelled broad beans
50g (2oz) low-fat soft cream cheese
4 eggs
2 tablespoons chopped thyme
freshly ground black pepper
2 tablespoons olive oil
1 onion, peeled and roughly chopped
225g (8oz) courgettes, sliced
125g (4oz) lightly cooked salmon, flaked

125g (4oz) cooked, peeled prawns

1. Cook the potatoes and broad beans separately in boiling water until just tender, then drain thoroughly.
2. In a bowl, whisk together the cheese, eggs, thyme and pepper.
3. Heat the oil in a large shallow ovenproof pan. Add the onion, courgettes, potatoes and beans. Cook, stirring, for 2–3 minutes.
4. Add the salmon and prawns and pour in the egg mixture. As the eggs cook, push the mixture to the centre to allow the raw egg to flow down the edge of the pan.

TURKEY SCHNITZEL
Serves 4

3 tbsp plain flour
seasoning
1 large egg, beaten
50g (2oz) fresh white breadcrumbs
4 x 175g (6oz) turkey breast escalopes

1. Sprinkle the flour onto a plate and season with a little salt and lots of black pepper. Pour the beaten egg onto another plate, and sprinkle the breadcrumbs onto a third plate.
2. Coat each escalope with the seasoned flour. Dip each floured escalope into the beaten egg, then dip into the breadcrumbs.
3. Cover and leave in the refrigerator for 30 minutes.
4. Bake in the oven for 30–40 minutes at 180°C/350°F/Gas 4 until the turkey is cooked through and the breadcrumbs are golden brown.

LAMB IN SPICY YOGHURT SAUCE

Serves 4

225ml (8floz) water
1tbsp olive oil
3 onions, sliced
900g (2lb) leg of lamb, boned and cut into 1.8cm (¾ inch)
    cubes
freshly ground black pepper
2 garlic cloves, crushed
1 tbsp fresh parsley
600ml (1 pint) natural bio yoghurt
1 tbsp cornflour, mixed to a paste with 2 tsp water
1 tsp grated lemon rind
1 tbsp chopped fresh coriander leaves

1. In a large saucepan, bring the water and oil to the boil
   over a moderate heat.
2. Add the onions, lamb, pepper, garlic and parsley. Cover
   the pan tightly, reduce the heat to low and simmer for 1¼
   hours or until the lamb is very tender and the liquid has
   reduced by about two-thirds of its original quantity.
3. In a medium saucepan, heat the yoghurt and cornflour
   mixture over a moderate heat, stirring constantly. Reduce
   the heat to very low and cook for 8 minutes until it has
   reduced by half its original quantity.
4. Add the yoghurt mixture and the lemon rind to the
   lamb mixture, stir well and simmer, uncovered, for 15
   minutes.
5. Add the coriander and serve with a crisp salad and boiled
   rice.

POTATO AND CHEESE BAKE
Serves 4

700g (1½ lb) potatoes, peeled
50g (2oz) margarine
2 medium onions, finely chopped
25g (1oz) flour
freshly ground black pepper to taste
½ tsp dried mixed herbs
350ml (12floz) milk
225g (8oz) Cheddar cheese, finely grated

1. Pre-heat the oven to 180°C (350F) Gas 4.
2. Boil and mash the potatoes. Place them in a medium mixing bowl and set aside.
3. Using a teaspoon of margarine, grease a medium ovenproof dish.
4. Melt the remaining margarine in a saucepan over a moderate heat. Add the onions and fry until softened and golden.
5. Remove the pan from the heat and with a wooden spoon stir in the flour, black pepper and herbs to make a smooth paste.
6. Gradually add the milk, stirring constantly and being careful to avoid lumps.
7. Return the pan to a low heat, stirring constantly, for 4–5 minutes or until the sauce is smooth and thick.
8. Add 175g (6oz) of the cheese and cook until it has melted, stirring all the time.
9. Gradually pour the cheese sauce over the potatoes, beating constantly with a wooden spoon until the mixture is smooth.
10. Turn the mixture into the prepared dish and smooth the mixture down with the back of a spoon. Sprinkle with the remaining cheese.
11. Place the dish in the centre of the oven and bake for 20–25 minutes or until the top is golden brown.
12. Serve immediately with broccoli and carrots.

OATY CHEESE QUICHE
Serves 4–6

Pastry
75g (3oz) self-raising flour
150g (5oz) fine oatmeal
freshly ground black pepper
125g (4oz) sunflower margarine
dried beans for baking 'blind'

Filling
350g (12oz) cottage cheese, sieved
30ml (2tbsp) natural yoghurt
6 sticks celery, chopped
75g (3oz) hazelnuts, chopped
pinch of curry powder

Garnish
pinch of paprika
tomato slices
parsley sprigs

1. Pre-heat the oven to 200°C (400°F) Gas 6.
2. Mix the flour and oatmeal together, with freshly ground pepper to taste. Cut in the margarine and rub in until the mixture resembles breadcrumbs. Stir in enough water to make a fairly stiff pastry and knead together lightly.
3. Turn on to a floured surface, roll out and use to line a 23cm (9 inch) flan ring. Cover the base with greaseproof paper and fill with dried beans. Bake 'blind' for 20 minutes. Remove the paper and beans and return the flan to the oven for 5 minutes. Allow to cool.
4. Mix the cheese, yoghurt, celery, nuts and curry powder together and pile into the flan case. Sprinkle with paprika and garnish with tomato and parsley.

BASIC WHITE SAUCE

25g (1oz) butter
25g (1oz) cornflour
300ml (½ pint) semi-skimmed milk
freshly ground sea salt and black pepper

1. Melt the butter in a small saucepan, then stir in the cornflour, stirring constantly until the mixture forms a smooth ball in the base of the saucepan.
2. Cook the flour mixture over a gently heat, stirring occasionally, for 2–3 minutes until it has a sandy texture, but has not changed colour. Allow to cool slightly before adding the liquid.
3. Gradually add the 300ml (½ pint) of hot milk to the cooked flour and butter mixture over a low heat, stirring until it is thick and smooth, then simmer gently, stirring occasionally, for 20 minutes. Season with black pepper and a little salt and a pinch of mustard powder if desired.
4. Use sauce for coating fish, and for cauliflower and broccoli cheese (see below).

Variations

Add a handful of freshly chopped parsley
Add 75g (3oz) grated mature Cheddar cheese or goats' cheese

CAULIFLOWER AND BROCCOLI CHEESE
Serves 4

1 medium size cauliflower
1 large head of broccoli
Basic white sauce (see above)
100g (4oz) mature Cheddar cheese, grated

1. Break the cauliflower and broccoli into florets and steam

until just tender, but not fully cooked. Put in a large
ovenproof dish.
2. Add half the grated cheese to some basic white sauce (see
page 277) and mix until all the cheese has melted.
3. Pour the cheese sauce over the broccoli and cauliflower,
then sprinkle the remaining cheese. Place in a hot oven
200°C/400°F/Gas 6 and cook for 30–40 minutes until
cooked through and golden brown on top.
4. Serve with extra fresh vegetables and jacket potato for a
hearty meal, or on its own for a lunch time snack.

DESSERTS – PHASE ONE

BAKED APPLE
Serves 1

1 cooking apple
1 dessertspoon of concentrated apple juice
1 cup of water
1 pinch of cinnamon

1. Wash and core the apple, and score around the centre of
the apple in a circle just breaking the skin.
2. Place the apple in an ovenproof dish.
3. Mix the concentrated apple juice with the water and the
cinnamon.
4. Pour the water into the dish, and pour the apple juice
over the apple.
5. Bake in a moderate oven 180°C/350°F/Gas 4 for
approximately 50–60 minutes.

BERRY TOFU CREAM
Serves 4

200g (7oz) firm tofu
200g (7oz) mixed berries (strawberries, raspberries,
    blueberries)
75g (3oz) ground almonds
1 pinch of cinnamon
2 tsp flaked, toasted almonds

1. Blend or process the tofu and berries together. To obtain
   a creamy texture, the mixture may need to be put through
   a sieve or food mill.
2. Add the ground almonds and mix well.
3. Spoon into 4 bowls or glasses and sprinkle lightly with the
   cinnamon and a few almond flakes.

CHRISTMAS PUDDING
Serves 8

1.2l (2 pint) pudding basin
2 eggs
125g (4oz) pure dairy free margarine
125g (4oz) alternative breadcrumbs (wheat, oats, rye and
    barley-free)
50g (2oz) brown rice flour
50g (2oz) corn flour
125g (4oz) molasses
1 large cooking apple, chopped
1 tsp cinnamon
1 tsp ginger
1 tsp mixed spice
225g (8oz) raisins
125g (4oz) sultanas
125g (4oz) currants
50g (2oz) mixed candied peel

1 grated carrot
50g (2oz) flaked almonds
zest of 1 large orange and lemon
3 tbsp rum
3 tbsp brandy
3 tbsp port
1 tsp baking powder (wheat free)
½ tsp bicarbonate of soda

1. Lightly grease the pudding basin.
2. Whisk the eggs and melt the margarine until soft.
3. Blend all the ingredients together and place in the pudding basin.
4. Cover with greaseproof paper and a layer of muslin or cotton. Tie with string and bring the sides of the muslin up and knot to make a handle which will make it easier to lift out of the pressure cooker when cooked.
5. Pressure cook for 2 hours for or until cooked through.

FRESH FRUIT SALAD

Serves 4

1 dessert apple, peeled and sliced
1 banana, peeled and sliced
60ml (4 tbsp) lemon juice
1 orange, peeled and segmented
1 grapefruit, peeled and segmented
125g (4oz) seedless grapes
2 kiwi fruit, peeled and sliced
30ml (2 tbsp) orange juice
4 sprigs of mint

1. Toss the apple and banana in the lemon juice. This will prevent discoloration.
2. Combine all fruits in a serving bowl, serve chilled and decorate with a sprig of mint.

CRANBERRY SORBET
Serves 4

300ml (½ pint) unsweetened orange juice
225g (8oz) fresh cranberries
300ml (½ pint) water
artificial sweetener to taste if necessary
2 egg whites

1. Place the orange juice and cranberries in a saucepan together with the water. Bring to the boil. Cover the saucepan and simmer gently for 2–3 minutes.
2. Strain the cranberries, keeping the cranberry juice in a separate bowl.
3. Blend the soft cranberries in a liquidiser and add the juices.
4. Allow to cool and add the sweetener, if necessary.
5. Put the cranberry mixture into a shallow dish and place in the freezer until semi-frozen.
6. Whisk the egg whites until stiff.
7. Remove the cranberry mixture from the freezer and break up the ice crystals that have formed.
8. Tip the semi-frozen sorbet into a bowl and fold in the whisked egg white.
9. Return the mixture to the container and freeze until firm.
10. When you are ready to serve, scoop the cranberry sorbet into decorative glasses.

DRIED FRUIT COMPÔTE
Serves 2

125g (4oz) mixture of dried fruits, e.g. peaches, prunes, apples, apricots and pears
75 ml (5 level tbsp) orange juice
2 whole cloves

2 x 2.5cm (1 inch) sticks cinnamon
juice and zest of ½ lemon

1. Wash the fruit and place it in a bowl with the orange
   juice, spices, lemon juice and zest.
2. Leave to soak overnight.
3. Next day, if the juice has been absorbed, add 2
   tablespoons of water. Then place the mixture in a
   saucepan, bring to the boil, cover and simmer on a very
   low heat for 10–15 minutes.
4. Transfer to a serving bowl, removing the cinnamon and
   cloves. Leave to cool or serve warm.

FRUIT SNOW
Serves 2

200g (7oz) dessert apples, peeled, cored and thinly sliced
30ml (2 tbsp) water
grated orange rind
1 large egg white, beaten until stiff
orange slices for garnish

1. Place apple, water and orange rind in a saucepan. Cover
   and cook gently, stirring occasionally until apples are soft.
2. Rub the apples through a sieve and let them cool.
3. Fold in the egg white and chill before serving. Serve with a
   slice of orange to decorate.

GLUTEN-FREE PANCAKES
Serves 4

125g (4oz) Dove's Farm gluten-free flour
1 small egg
300ml (½ pint) skimmed soya or rice milk

1. Make a thin batter with the flour, egg and milk.

2. Use kitchen paper to wipe a small non-stick frying pan with a little oil and heat until the oil is smoking.
3. Pour a generous 30ml (2 tablespoons) of batter into the pan and swirl it around to cover the base. Cook for 60 seconds.
4. Flip the pancake over and cook for a further few seconds.

PEACH SUNDAE

Serves 2

2 peaches
150g (5oz) raspberries
2½ tsp sugar
1 tsp arrowroot
2 tsp shredded, or toasted, desiccated coconut

1. Skin the peaches by blanching them. (Pour boiling water over them, leave to cool briefly, and then place in cold water. The skins will then peel off easily).
2. Halve the peaches and remove the stones.
3. Sieve the raspberries, making a purée.
4. Take a little of the raspberry purée and mix with the sugar and arrowroot into a paste.
5. Stir the arrowroot paste into the raspberry purée, and add sugar.
6. Place the mixture in a saucepan and boil for 1 minute, stirring constantly.
7. When the mixture has cooled, pour the sauce over the peaches and sprinkle with the coconut.

GLUTEN-FREE PASTRY

125g (4oz) Dove's Farm gluten-free flour
1 egg
50g (2oz) pure margarine

1. Combine all the ingredients and form into a small ball.
2. Roll out on to greaseproof paper.
3. To keep pastry intact, place a flan dish face down on to the greaseproof paper and invert it. Lightly press the pastry down and around the sides of the flan dish. Fill and bake as directed, depending on which recipe is used for the filling.

DESSERTS – PHASE TWO

TROPICAL CRUMBLE
Serves 4

4 bananas, sliced
2 tbsp brown sugar
2 tbsp pure maple syrup
50g (2oz) rice flour
50g (2oz) porridge oats
25g (1oz) soft brown sugar
15g (1½ tsp) desiccated coconut
50g (2oz) butter, melted

1. Place the sliced bananas, sugar and maple syrup in an ovenproof dish and cook under a low grill for 3 minutes.
2. Mix the dry ingredients together and pour over the melted butter.
3. Sprinkle the oaty topping over the bananas and grill under a moderate heat for a further 3 minutes, until golden brown and crunchy.
4. Serve with custard or ice-cream.

Note: This topping works very well with any type of fresh fruit.

YOGHURT ICE-CREAM
Serves 4

225g (8oz) raspberries, plums, peaches or other soft fruit
275g (10oz) natural yoghurt
5ml (1 tsp) concentrated apple juice to sweeten
mint sprig to decorate

1. Wash and prepare the fruit as necessary, and purée it in the liquidiser with the apple juice.
2. Place the mixture in the freezer for 2–3 hours until semi-frozen.
3. Remove the mixture from the freezer, add the yoghurt and whisk well, then freeze until firm.
4. Place the yoghurt ice-cream in the refrigerator 30 minutes before serving to allow it to soften.
5. Scoop the ice-cream into chilled dessert dishes and decorate with fruit or mint.

BANANA AND TOFU CREAM
Serves 4

200g (7oz) firm tofu
200g (7oz) bananas, skinned
75g (3oz) ground almonds
1 pinch of cinnamon
2 tsp almond flakes

1. Blend or process the tofu and bananas together. To obtain a creamy texture, the mixture may need to be put through a sieve or food mill.
2. Add the ground almonds and mix well.
3. Spoon into 4 bowls or glasses and sprinkle lightly with cinnamon and almond flakes.

MELON ICE-CREAM
Serves 4

1 medium melon (Ogen or similar if you can get it)
300ml (½ pint) plain yoghurt
concentrated apple juice to sweeten if necessary
16 raspberries to decorate

1. Halve the melon, scoop out the seeds and then scoop out the melon flesh and place in the liquidiser.
2. Liquidise the melon flesh and mix with the yoghurt and concentrated apple juice as needed.
3. Place the melon and yoghurt mixture in a shallow dish and freeze until firm.
4. Scoop the melon ice-cream into dessert glasses and decorate with raspberries.

GRAPEFRUIT SORBET
Serves 4

2 grapefruits
450ml (¾ pint) water
concentrated apple juice
45ml (3 tbsp) natural yoghurt
2 egg whites
peeled grapefruit segments for decoration

1. Thinly pare the rind from the grapefruit and place the grapefruit rind and water into a pan. Simmer gently for 8 minutes and strain into a bowl.
2. Cut the fruit in half and squeeze out the juice.
3. Add the grapefruit juice to the liquid from the grapefuit rind into a bowl and add apple juice to taste.
4. Pour the grapefruit liquid into a shallow freezer container and freeze until semi-frozen.
5. Turn the semi-frozen grapefruit mixture into a bowl and

beat to break up the ice crystals.
6. Mix in the yoghurt.
7. Whisk the egg white until stiff and fold into the grapefruit and yoghurt mixture gently.
8. Return to the freezer until firm.
9. Scoop out the sorbet into dessert glasses and decorate with peeled grapefruit segments.

CAKES AND BISCUITS – PHASE ONE AND TWO

CRUNCHY SEED SQUARES
Makes 8 slices

3 tbsp brown rice syrup
1 tbsp honey
7 tbsp walnut oil
75g (3oz) porridge oats*
75g (3oz) soya flour
2 tbsp ground almonds
1 tbsp sunflower seeds
1 tbsp pumpkin seeds
1 tbsp linseeds
50g (2oz) flaked almonds

1. Warm the brown rice syrup, honey and walnut oil and mix thoroughly with the dry ingredients.
2. Press into a greased 9" x 9" square cake tin and bake in a preheated oven at 180°C/350°F/Gas 4 for 25 minutes.

Note: Use buckwheat flakes or Dove's Farm gluten-free flour for a totally wheat- and gluten-free version. Add a little more syrup and oil if the mixture appears too dry.

GLUTEN-FREE SCONES
Makes 6

50g (2oz) rice flour
50g (2oz) buckwheat flour
125g (4oz) potato flour
50g (2oz) ground almonds or soya flour
1 dstp baking powder
50g (2oz) butter or margarine
50g (2oz) caster sugar
150ml (¼ pint) soya milk
1 egg beaten

1. Combine the flours and baking powder in a large bowl.
2. Add the butter or margarine and mix with fingertips until it resembles fine breadcrumbs.
3. Stir in the sugar, soya milk and beaten egg and mix well.
4. The mixture will be fairly moist, so if you cannot roll it out, just place spoonfuls onto a baking tray. Brush the tops with soya milk.
5. Bake at 200°C/425°F/Gas 7 for 10–15 minutes until golden brown.

Variations
Cheese scones
Add 100g (4oz) grated Cheddar cheese
1 tsp mustard powder
1 dstp mixed herbs

Fruit scones
100g (4oz) mixed dried fruit

Sugar free scones
Omit the sugar and serve with nut butters and sugar free fruit spreads

NUTTY FRUIT TEA LOAF

Serves 8

375g (12oz) mixed dried fruit
juice and rind of 1 lemon
300ml (½ pint) strong, hot redbush tea
75g (3oz) whole almonds
75g (3oz) pecan nuts
300g (10oz) Dove's Farm gluten-free flour
1 tsp ground mixed spice
1 tsp ground ginger
3 tsp baking powder
1 egg, beaten
soya milk

1. Combine the dried fruit with the lemon juice and rind in a large bowel and leave to soak in the hot redbush tea for at least 8 hours.
2. Toast the nuts until lightly golden and leave to cool.
3. Put the Dove's Farm flour into a separate bowl with the spices and baking powder, then combine thoroughly with the toasted nuts, soaked fruit and remaining liquid. Add the egg and stir well. If the mixture appears too dry, add a few tablespoons of soya milk.
4. Line a 900g (2lb) loaf tin, and put the tea loaf mixture in, roughly smoothing the top. Bake at 150°C/300°F/Gas 2 for approximately 1½ – 1⅓ hours, or until well risen and firm to touch.
5. Serve cold, or lightly toasted with pure fruit jam or cheese.

ALMOND MACAROONS

Makes 18 biscuits

2 large egg whites
150g (6oz) ground almonds
75g (3oz) unrefined caster sugar
18 almonds halves

1. Put the unbeaten egg whites into a large bowl with the ground almonds. Beat well adding the caster sugar 1 tablespoon at a time.
2. Line biscuit trays with greaseproof paper.
3. Roll the mixture into balls and flatten with the palm of your hand.
4. Lay the flattened biscuits onto the trays and place an almond half in the middle of each biscuit.
5. Bake in a moderate oven at 180°C/350°F/Gas 4 for 25 minutes or until golden brown.

COCONUT PYRAMIDS

Makes 24

4 egg yolks or 2 whole eggs
75g (3oz) unrefined caster sugar
juice and rind of half a lemon
250g (8oz) desiccated coconut

1. Beat the eggs and sugar until creamy.
2. Stir in the lemon juice, rind and coconut.
3. Form into pyramid shapes either with your hands or using a moist egg cup and place on a greased baking tray.
4. Bake at 190°C/375°F/Gas 5 for 20–25 minutes until the tips are golden brown.

LEMON AND ALMOND CAKE

170g (6oz) pure dairy-free margarine
150g (5oz) unrefined caster sugar
3 eggs
170g (6oz) Dove's Farm gluten-free flour
50g (2oz) ground almonds
grated rind and juice of 1 lemon
½ teaspoon almond essence

To finish
2 lemons
2 tablespoons clear honey

1. Preheat the oven to 160°/325°F/Gas 3. Grease and line an 8-inch loose-bottomed round cake tin.
2. Place the cake ingredients in a large bowl and mix well. Beat with a wooden spoon or electric whisk for 2–3 minutes until light and fluffy.
3. Turn mixture into the cake tin and smooth the top. Pare the rind and pith of the two lemons, then slice into thin round slices and place on top of the cake.
4. Bake for 50–60 minutes until golden and firm. Cool in tin for 10 minutes, then release the sides and cool on a wire rack. Warm the honey and brush over the cake and serve.

SIMPLY SMOOTHIES – PHASE ONE

BANANA AND MIXED SUMMER BERRY SMOOTHIE
Serves 2

2 medium bananas
125g (4oz) frozen summer berries (raspberries, strawberries, redcurrants, blueberries)
300ml (½ pint) ice-cold soya milk

1. Put all the ingredients into a blender or process with a hand blender, pour into glasses and serve.

Note: Frozen berries are better than fresh as they make a thicker, icier consistency and very often they contain more nutrients.

TROPICAL MANGO
Serves 2

1 medium mango
2 bananas
300ml (½ pint) soya or cows' milk
150ml (¼ pint) coconut milk

1. Peel and chop the mango and bananas and combine with the ice-cold milk. Put all the ingredients into a blender and whizz until smooth. Add more milk to adjust the consistency.

MIXED BERRY SMOOTHIE
Serves 2

250g (8oz) frozen or fresh mixed summer berries (raspberries, strawberries, blueberries, blackcurrants)
450ml (¾ pint) ice-cold soya milk
4 tbsp strawberry soya yoghurt

1. Combine all the ingredients and blend until smooth. Add more soya milk according to taste.

PART **FOUR**

THE MODEL PLAN
IN ACTION

Nutritional content of food lists

Unless stated otherwise, foods listed are raw

Vitamin A – retinol
Micrograms per 100g (3.5oz)

Skimmed milk	1
Semi-skimmed milk	21
Grilled herring	49
Whole milk	52
Porridge made with milk	56
Cheddar cheese	325
Margarine	800
Butter	815
Lamb's liver	15,000

Vitamin B1 – thiamin
Milligrams per 100g (3.5oz)

Peaches	0.02
Cottage cheese	0.02
Cox's apple	0.03
Full-fat milk	0.04
Skimmed milk	0.04
Semi-skimmed milk	0.04
Cheddar cheese	0.04
Bananas	0.04
White grapes	0.04
French beans	0.04
Low-fat yogurt	0.05
Canteloupe melon	0.05
Tomato	0.06
Green peppers, raw	0.0?
Boiled egg	0.08
Roast chicken	0.08
Grilled cod	0.08
Haddock, steamed	0.08
Roast turkey	0.09
Mackerel, cooked	0.09
Savoy cabbage, boiled	0.10
Oranges	0.10
Brussels sprouts	0.10
Lentils, boiled	0.11
Potatoes, new, boiled	0.11
Soya beans, boiled	0.12
Red peppers, raw	0.12
Steamed salmon	0.20
Corn	0.20
White spaghetti, boiled	0.21
Almonds	0.24
White self-raising flour	0.30
Plaice, steamed	0.30
Bacon, cooked	0.35
Walnuts	0.40
Wholemeal flour	0.47
Lamb's kidney	0.49
Brazil nuts	1.00
Cornflakes	1.00
Rice Krispies	1.00
Wheatgerm	2.01

Vitamin B2 – riboflavin
Milligrams per 100g (3.5oz)

Cabbage, boiled	0.01
Potatoes, boiled	0.01
Brown rice, boiled	0.02
Pear	0.03
Wholemeal spaghetti, boiled	0.03
White self-raising flour	0.03
Orange	0.04
Spinach, boiled in salted water	0.05
Baked beans	0.06
Banana	0.06
White bread	0.06
Green peppers, raw	0.08
Lentils, boiled	0.08
Hovis	0.09
Soya beans, boiled	0.09
Wholemeal bread	0.09
Wholemeal flour	0.09

Peanuts	0.10	Red peppers, raw	2.20
Baked salmon	0.11	Almonds	3.10
Red peppers, raw	0.15	Grilled herring	4.00
Full-fat milk	0.17	Wholemeal bread	4.10
Avocado	0.18	Hovis	4.20
Grilled herring	0.18	Wholemeal flour	5.70
Semi-skimmed milk	0.18	Muesli	6.50
Roast chicken	0.19	Topside of beef, cooked	*6.50*
Roast turkey	0.21	Leg of lamb, cooked	6.60
Cottage cheese	0.26	Baked salmon	7.00
Soya flour	031	Roast chicken	8.20
Boiled prawns	0.34	Roast turkey	8.50
Boiled egg	0.35	Boiled prawns	9.50
Topside of beef, cooked	*0.35*	Peanuts	13.80
Leg of lamb, cooked	0.38	Cornflakes	16.00
Cheddar cheese	0.40	Rice Krispies	16.00
Muesli	0.70		
Almonds	*0.75*		
Cornflakes	1.50		
Rice Krispies	1.50		

Vitamin B3 – niacin

Vitamin B6 – pyridoxine

Milligrams per 100g (3.5oz)

Milligrams per 100g (3.5oz)		Carrots	*0.05*
		Full-fat milk	0.06
Boiled egg	0.07	Skimmed milk	0.06
Cheddar cheese	0.07	Semi-skimmed milk	0.06
Full-fat milk	0.08	Satsuma	0.07
Skimmed milk	0.09	White bread	0.07
Semi-skimmed milk	0.09	White rice	0.07
Cottage cheese	0.13	Cabbage, boiled	0.08
Cox's apple	0.20	Cottage cheese	0.08
Cabbage, boiled	0.30	Cox's apple	0.08
Orange	0.40	Wholemeal pasta	0.08
Baked beans	0.50	Frozen peas	0.08
Potatoes, boiled	0.50	Spinach, boiled	0.09
Soya beans, boiled	0.50	Cheddar cheese	0.10
Lentils, boiled	0.60	Orange	0.10
Banana	0.70	Broccoli	0.11
Tomato	1.00	Hovis	0.11
Avocado	1.10	Baked beans	0.12
Green peppers, raw	1.10	Boiled egg	0.12
Brown rice	1.30	Red kidney beans, cooked	0.12
Wholemeal spaghetti, boiled	1.30	Wholemeal bread	0.12
White self-raising flour	1.50	Tomatoes	0.14
Grilled cod	1.70	Almonds	0.15
White bread	1.70	Cauliflower	0.15
Soya flour	2.00	Brussels sprouts	0.19
		Sweetcorn, boiled	0.21
		Leg of lamb, cooked	0.22

Grapefruit juice	0.23
Roast chicken	0.26
Lentils, boiled	0.28
Banana	0.29
Brazil nuts	0.31
Potatoes, boiled	0.32
Roast turkey	0.33
Grilled herring	0.33
Topside of beef, cooked	0.33
Avocado	0.36
Grilled cod	0.38
Baked salmon	0.57
Soya flour	0.57
Hazelnuts	0.59
Peanuts	0.59
Walnuts	0.67
Muesli	1.60
Cornflakes	1.80
Rice Krispies	1.80
Special K	2.20

Vitamin B12
Micrograms per 100g (3.5oz)

Tempeh	0.10
Miso	0.20
Quorn	0.30
Full-fat milk	0.40
Skimmed milk	0.40
Semi-skimmed milk	0.40
Marmite	0.50
Cottage cheese	0.70
Choux buns	1.00
Eggs, boiled	1.00
Eggs, poached	1.00
Halibut, steamed	1.00
Lobster, boiled	1.00
Sponge cake	1.00
Turkey, white meat	1.00
Waffles	1.00
Cheddar cheese	1.20
Eggs, scrambled	1.20
Squid, fresh	1.30
Eggs, fried	1.60
Shrimps, boiled	1.80
Parmesan cheese	1.90
Beef, lean	2.00
Cod, baked	2.00
Cornflakes	2.00
Pork, cooked	2.00
Raw beef mince	2.00
Rice Krispies	2.00
Steak, lean, grilled	2.00
Edam cheese	2.10
Eggs, whole, battery	2.40
Milk, dried, whole	2.40
Milk, dried, skimmed	2.60
Eggs, whole, free-range	2.70
Kambu seaweed	2.80
Squid, frozen	2.90
Taramasalata	2.90
Duck, cooked	3.00
Turkey, dark meat	3.00
Grapenuts	5.00
Tuna in oil	5.00
Herring, cooked	6.00
Herring roe, fried	6.00
Steamed salmon	6.00
Bovril	8.30
Mackerel, fried	10.00
Rabbit, stewed	10.00
Cod's roe, fried	11.00
Pilchards canned in tomato juice	12.00
Oysters, raw	15.00
Nori seaweed	27.50
Sardines in oil	28.00
Lamb's kidney, fried	79.00

Folate/Folic acid
Micrograms per 100g (3.5oz)

Cox's apple	4.00
Leg of lamb, cooked	4.00
Full-fat milk	6.00
Skimmed milk	6.00
Semi-skimmed milk	6.00
Porridge with semi-skimmed milk	7.00
Turnip, baked	8.00
Sweet potato, boiled	8.00
Cucumber	9.00
Grilled herring	10.00
Roast chicken	10.00

Avocado	11.00	Hazelnuts	72.00
Grilled cod	12.00	Spinach, boiled	90.00
Banana	14.00	Brussels sprouts	110.00
Roast turkey	15.00	Peanuts	110.00
Carrots	17.00	Muesli	140.00
Sweet potato	17.00	Sweetcorn, boiled	150.00
Tomatoes	17.00	Asparagus	155.00
Topside of beef, cooked	17.00	Chickpeas	180.00
Swede, boiled	18.00	Lamb's liver, fried	240.00
Strawberries	20.00	Cornflakes	250.00
Brazil nuts	21.00	Rice Krispies	250.00
Red peppers, raw	21.00	Calves' liver, fried	320.00
Green peppers, raw	23.00		
Rye bread	24.00	**Vitamin C**	
Dates, fresh	25.00	*Milligrams per 100g (3.5oz)*	
New potatoes, boiled	25.00	Full-fat milk	1.00
Grapefruit	26.00	Skimmed milk	1.00
Oatcakes	26.00	Semi-skimmed milk	1.00
Cottage cheese	27.00	Red kidney beans	1.00
Baked salmon	29.00	Carrots	2.00
Cabbage, boiled	29.00	Cucumber	2.00
Onions, boiled	29.00	Muesli with dried fruit	2.00
White bread	29.00	Apricots, raw	6.00
Orange	31.00	Avocado	6.00
Baked beans	33.00	Pear	6.00
Cheddar cheese	33.00	Potato, boiled	6.00
Clementines	33.00	Spinach, boiled	8.00
Raspberries	33.00	Cox's apple	9.00
Satsuma	33.00	Turnip	10.00
Blackberries	34.00	Banana	11.00
Rye crispbread	35.00	Frozen peas	12.00
Potato, baked in skin	36.00	Lamb's liver, fried	12.00
Radish	38.00	Pineapple	12.00
Boiled egg	39.00	Dried skimmed milk	13.00
Hovis	39.00	Gooseberries	14.00
Wholemeal bread	39.00	Raw dates	14.00
Red kidney beans, boiled	42.00	Melon	17.00
Potato, baked	44.00	Tomatoes	17.00
Frozen peas	47.00	Cabbage, boiled	20.00
Almonds	48.00	Canteloupe melon	26.00
Parsnips, boiled	48.00	Cauliflower	27.00
Cauliflower	51.00	Satsuma	27.00
Green beans, boiled	57.00	Peach	31.00
Broccoli	64.00	Raspberries	32.00
Walnuts	66.00	Bran flakes	35.00
Artichoke	68.00	Grapefruit	36.00

Mangoes	37.00	Cheddar cheese	0.53
Nectarine	37.00	Carrots	0.56
Kumquats	39.00	Lettuce	0.57
Broccoli	44.00	Cox's apple	0.59
Lychees	45.00	Grilled cod	0.59
Unsweetened apple juice	49.00	Rice Krispies	0.60
Orange	54.00	Plums	0.61
Kiwi fruit	59.00	Unsweetened orange juice	0.68
Brussels sprouts	60.00	Leeks	0.78
Strawberries	77.00	Sweetcorn, boiled	0.88
Blackcurrants	115.00	Brussels sprouts	0.90
		Broccoli	1.10
		Boiled egg	1.11

Vitamin D
Micrograms per 100g (3.5oz)

Skimmed milk	0.01	Tomato	1.22
Whole milk	0.03	Watercress	1.46
Fromage frais	0.05	Parsley	1.70
Cheddar cheese	0.26	Spinach, boiled	1.71
Cornflakes	2.80	Olives	1.99
Rice Krispies	2.80	Butter	2.00
Kellogg's Start	4.20	Onions, dried raw	2.69
Margarine	8.00	Mushrooms, fried in corn oil	2.84
		Avocado	3.20
		Muesli	3.20

Vitamin E
Milligrams per 100g (3.5oz)

		Walnuts	3.85
Semi-skimmed milk	0.03	Peanut butter	4.99
Boiled potatoes	0.06	Olive oil	5.10
Cucumber	0.07	Sweet potato, baked	5.96
Cottage cheese	0.08	Brazil nuts	7.18
Full-fat milk	0.09	Peanuts	10.09
Cabbage, boiled	0.10	Pine nuts	13.65
Leg of lamb, cooked	0.10	Rapeseed oil	18.40
Cauliflower	0.11	Almonds	23.96
Roast chicken	0.11	Hazelnuts	24.98
Frozen peas	0.18	Sunflower oil	48.70
Red kidney beans, cooked	0.20		
Wholemeal bread	0.20	**Calcium**	

Milligrams per 100 g(3.5oz)

Orange	2.4	Cox's apple	4.00
Topside of beef, cooked	0.26	Brown rice, boiled	4.00
Banana	0.27	Potatoes, boiled	5.00
Brown rice, boiled	0.30	Banana	6.00
Grilled herring	0.30	Topside of beef, cooked	6.00
Lamb's liver, fried	0.32	White pasta, boiled	7.00
Baked beans	0.36	Tomato	7.00
Cornflakes	0.40	White spaghetti, boiled	7.00
Pear	0.50	Leg of lamb, cooked	8.00

Red peppers, raw	8.00
Roast chicken	9.00
Roast turkey	9.00
Avocado	11.00
Pear	11.00
Butter	15.00
Cornflakes	15.00
White rice, boiled	18.00
Grilled cod	22.00
Lentils, boiled	22.00
Baked salmon	29.00
Green peppers, raw	30.00
Young carrots	30.00
Grilled herring	33.00
Wholemeal flour	38.00
Turnips, baked	45.00
Orange	47.00
Baked beans	48.00
Wholemeal bread	54.00
Boiled egg	57.00
Peanuts	60.00
Cottage cheese	73.00
Soya beans, boiled	83.00
White bread	100.00
Full-fat milk	115.00
Hovis	120.00
Muesli	120.00
Skimmed milk	120.00
Semi-skimmed milk	120.00
Prawns, boiled	150.00
Spinach, boiled	150.00
Brazil nuts	170.00
Yoghurt, low-fat, plain	190.00
Soya flour	210.00
Almonds	240.00
White self-raising flour	4.50.00
Sardines	550.00
Sprats, fried	710.00
Cheddar cheese	720.00
Whitebait, fried	860.00

Chromium
Milligrams per 100g (3.5oz)

Milk	1
Cabbage	4
Green beans	4

Mushrooms	4
Orange	5
Lettuce	7
Shrimps	7
Carrots	9
Banana	10
Spinach	10
Scallops	11
Butter	13
Parsnips	13
Apple	14
Hens' eggs	16
Green (bell) peppers	19
Pork chops	20
Potatoes	24
Fresh chilli	30
Rye bread	30
Lamb chops	42
Chicken	45
Calves' liver	55
Brewer's yeast	112

Iron
Milligrams per 100g (3.5oz)

Semi-skimmed milk	0.05
Skimmed milk	0.06
Full-fat milk	0.06
Cottage cheese	0.10
Orange	0.10
Cox's apple	0.20
Pear	0.20
White rice	0.20
Banana	0.30
Cabbage, boiled	0.30
Cheddar cheese	0.30
Avocado	0.40
Grilled cod	0.40
Potatoes, boiled	0.40
Young carrots, boiled	0.40
Brown rice, boiled	0.50
Tomato	0.50
White pasta, boiled	0.50
Baked salmon	0.80
Roast chicken	0.80
Roast turkey	0.90
Grilled herring	1.00

Red peppers, raw	1.00	Topside of beef, cooked	24.00
Boiled prawns	1.10	White bread	24.00
Green peppers, raw	1.20	Avocado	25.00
Baked beans	1.40	Cheddar cheese	25.00
Wholemeal spaghetti, boiled	1.40	Grilled cod	26.00
White bread	1.60	Roast turkey	27.00
Spinach, boiled	1.70	Leg of lamb, cooked	28.00
Boiled egg	1.90	Baked salmon	29.00
White self-raising flour	2.00	Baked beans	31.00
Brazil nuts	2.50	Spinach, boiled	31.00
Peanuts	2.50	Grilled herring	32.00
Leg of lamb, cooked	2.70	Banana	34.00
Wholemeal bread	2.70	Lentils, boiled	34.00
Topside of beef, cooked	2.80	Boiled prawns	42.00
Almonds	3.00	Wholemeal spaghetti, boiled	42.00
Soya beans, boiled	3.00	Brown rice, boiled	43.00
Lentils, boiled	3.50	Hovis	56.00
Hovis	3.70	Soya beans, boiled	63.00
Wholemeal flour	3.90	Wholemeal bread	76.00
Muesli	5.60	Muesli	85.00
Cornflakes	6.70	Wholemeal flour	120.00
Rice Krispies	6.70	Peanuts	210.00
Soya flour	6.90	Soya flour	240.00
		Almonds	270.00
		Brazil nuts	410.00

Magnesium
Milligrams per 100g (3.5oz)

Selenium
Micrograms per 100g (3.5oz)

Butter	2.00		
Cox's apple	6.00	Full-fat milk	1.00
Turnip, baked	6.00	Semi-skimmed milk	1.00
Young carrots	6.00	Skimmed milk	1.00
Tomato	7.00	Baked beans	2.00
Cottage cheese	9.00	Cornflakes	2.00
Orange	10.00	Orange	2.00
Full-fat milk	11.00	Peanuts	3.00
White rice, boiled	11.00	Almonds	4.00
Semi-skimmed milk	11.00	Cottage cheese	4.00
Skimmed milk	12.00	White rice	4.00
Boiled egg	12.00	White self-raising flour	4.00
Cornflakes	14.00	Soya beans, boiled	5.00
Potatoes, boiled	14.00	Boiled egg	11.00
Red peppers, raw	14.00	Cheddar cheese	12.00
White pasta	15.00	White bread	28.00
White spaghetti, boiled	15.00	Wholemeal bread	35.00
White self-raising flour	20.00	Lentils, boiled	40.00
Green peppers, raw	24.00	Wholemeal flour	53.00
Roast chicken	24.00		

Zinc

Milligrams per 100g (3.5oz)

Butter	0.10
Pear	0.10
Orange	0.10
Red peppers, raw	0.10
Banana	0.20
Young carrots	0.20
Cornflakes	0.30
Potatoes, boiled	0.30
Avocado	0.40
Full-fat milk	0.40
Skimmed milk	0.40
Green peppers, raw	0.40
Semi-skimmed milk	0.40
Baked beans	0.50
Grilled cod	0.50
Grilled herring	0.50
White pasta	0.50
Tomatoes	0.50
Cottage cheese	0.60
Spinach, boiled	0.60
White bread	0.60
White self-raising flour	0.60
Brown rice	0.70
White rice	0.70
Soya beans, boiled	0.90
Wholemeal spaghetti, boiled	1.10
Boiled egg	1.30
Lentils, boiled	1.40
Roast chicken	1.50
Boiled prawns	1.60
Wholemeal bread	1.80
Hovis	2.10
Cheddar cheese	2.30
Roast turkey	2.40
Muesli	2.50
Wholemeal flour	2.90
Almonds	3.20
Peanuts	3.50
Brazil nuts	4.20
Leg of lamb, cooked	5.30
Topside of beef, cooked	5.50

Essential fatty acids

Exact amounts of these fats are hard to quantify. Good sources for the two families of essential fatty acids are given.

Omega-6 series essential fatty acids

Sunflower oil
Rapeseed oil
Corn oil
Almonds
Walnuts
Brazil nuts
Sunflower seeds
Soya products including tofu

Omega-3 series essential fatty acids

Mackerel ⎫
Herring ⎬ fresh cooked or smoked/pickled
Salmon ⎭
Walnuts and walnut oil
Rapeseed oil
Soya products and soya bean oil

Healthy shopping options

PHASE I

SUITABLE FOR PHASE ONE OF THE DISCOVERY DIET AND HEALTHY EATING PLAN

CEREALS
Cornflakes
Puffed rice
Wake-up muesli
Rice Krispies

PASTA AND GRAINS
Brown rice
Buckwheat
Rice noodles
Corn pasta
Rice pasta
Buckwheat noodles

DAIRY ALTERNATIVES
Soya milk, Granose, SoGood, Provamel, Plamil
Heinz organic and vanilla soya milk
Provamel 'Soya Dream'
Provamel 'Soya Fruity'
Provamel Yofu – natural and fruit
Granose soya margarine
Tofutti 'cream cheese'
Swedish Glace 'ice-cream'
Oatly (oat 'milk')
Evernat almond and hazelnut 'milk'
'Pure' soya margarine

BREAD ALTERNATIVES
Barkat white or brown rice bread
Village Bakery Chestnut gluten-free bread
Corn crispbread (Orgran)

Rice crispbread (Orgran)
Rice cakes
Corn cakes
Glutano gluten-free crackers
Quaker Corn and rice cakes
Uncle Ben's Rispinos

BEVERAGES
Fruit juice (organic where possible) and other pure fruit juices
Amé
Aqua Libra
James White organic fruit juices
Redbush or Rooibos herbal tea 'look-alike'
Fruit tea
Dandelion coffee
Irish Spring lightly carbonated fruit water
Innocent smoothies
Pete and Johnny smoothies

MISCELLANEOUS/SNACKS
Dove's Farm gluten-free flour mix
Chick pea flour
Soya flour
Dove's Farm gluten-free lemon cookies
Wake-up bar
Sesame seed bars
Granny Ann gluten-free cookies
Rite Diet/Glutafin biscuits
Japanese rice crackers
Kettle crisps
Poppadums

SUITABLE FOR PHASE ONE AND TWO OF THE DISCOVERY DIET AND HEALTHY EATING PLAN

NUTS, SEEDS AND DRIED FRUIT
Linusit Gold linseeds
Pumpkin seeds
Sunflower seeds
Sesame seeds
Dried apricots

Raisins
Sultanas
Pine kernels
Soya flakes
Pecan nuts
Almonds – whole and ground

PULSES
Chick peas
Kidney beans
Lentils – brown, red, puy
Soya beans
Mixed beans
Baked beans

SPREADS
Meridian pure fruit spread – strawberry, black cherry, apricot,
    marmalade
Whole Earth pure fruit spread
Nut 'butter' – almond, hazelnut, peanut, cashew
St Dalfour 100 per cent fruit spreads
Yeo Valley fruit compôte

VEGETARIAN PROTEIN
Tofu
Quorn
Veggie sausages and burgers (free from forbidden ingredients)
Falafel (chick pea patties)
Hoummos
Eggs
Dahl

FISH AND POULTRY
Oily fish including mackerel, pilchards, salmon, sardines, herring
White fish, cod, haddock, plaice
Prawns
Chicken
Turkey
Game
Lamb
Lean beef
Steak mince

FRUIT AND VEGETABLES
Variety of fresh fruit – kiwis, apples, pears, bananas, etc
Variety of fresh salad ingredients
Selection of fresh vegetables particularly green leafy – broccoli,
    spinach, curly kale
Potatoes

PHASE TWO

SUITABLE FOR PHASE TWO OF THE DISCOVERY DIET AND HEALTHY EATING PLAN

CEREALS
Porridge oats
Shredded Wheat
Weetabix
Jordan's Oat Crunchy cereal

PASTA AND GRAINS
Couscous
Bulgar wheat
Wholewheat
White pasta
Wholewheat pasta
Gnocchi
Ravioli
Tortellini

BREAD & CRACKERS
Waitrose 100 per cent organic sliced rye bread
Village Bakery 100 per cent rye bread
Nairn's Oatcakes
Terence Stamp wheat-free bread with sunflower or poppy seeds
Finn Crisp rye crispbread
Dove's Farm rye crackers
Ryvita
White bread
Wholemeal/granary bread
Bagels
Muffins

French bread (100 per cent French flour)
Ciabatta
Pitta

DAIRY
Yeo Valley natural bio yoghurt
Yeo Valley bio yoghurt assorted flavours
Yeo Valley crème fraîche
Goats' cheese
Feta
Mozzarella
Edam
Cottage cheese
Tzatziki

BEVERAGES
Whole Earth NoCaf cereal alternative to coffee
Barley Cup
Caro

MISCELLANEOUS/SNACKS
Terence Stamp all purpose wheat-free flour
Terence Stamp wheat-free pasta mix
Terence Stamp wheat-free soda bread mix
Wake-up bar
DeRit honey rye cake
Village Bakery Trophy Bars (wheat-free)
Jordan's cereal bars
Flapjacks
Wholewheat digestives
Scones – fruit and cheese

Good food – where to find it?

This is a useful guide to where you can buy wholesome foods to eat whilst following the Discovery Diet and Healthy Eating Plan. However, the directory is subject to change, as new products are being developed even as the book goes to print!

Baker Bennetts Ltd

14 St Chads House, School Lane, Rochdale, Lancashire OL16 1QU. Tel: 01706 650356, email: bakerbennetts@dial.pipex.com

Manufacturers of rye and wheat crispbreads, made from natural ingredients, sold under the name of Finn Crisp. Available from all major supermarkets.

Harvest wheat
Original rye
Finn Crisp traditional
Finn Crisp multigrain
Organic crisp bread

Buxton Foods Ltd

12 Harley Street, London W1G 9PG,
Tel: 0207 6375505, email: k.towers@stamp-collection.co.uk,
www.stamp-collection.co.uk

Rapid growth for Buxton Foods, sold under the name Terence Stamp Collection in the special dietary foods market. Most major supermarkets stock selected lines, however, Sainsburys is the first supermarket to stock the complete range. The Stamp Collection was pioneered by Terence Stamp, who suffers himself with cow's milk and wheat intolerance. All products in the range are free from wheat and cow's milk.

All purpose wheat free flour
Bread
Sliced bread
Pasta and soda bread mixes
Fresh pasta
Sheep's milk cheese

Cauldron Foods

Units 1-2, Portishead Business Park, Portishead, Bristol BS20 7BF.
Tel: 01275 818448, www.cauldronfoods.co.uk

Innovative range of delicious vegetarian and organic convenience
foods. Available from all major supermarkets and health food stores.
All products are suitable for a vegetarian diet.

Glamorgan sausages
Falafel
Nut cutlets
Bean burgers
Nut roast
Pate
Tofu/marinated tofu

Clipper Teas

Beaminster Business Park, Broadwindsor Road, Beaminster, Dorset
DT8 3PR.
Tel 01308 863344, email simon@clipper-teas.com,
www.clipper.teas.com

Winners of ten organic awards, Clipper provides delicious varieties
of tea and coffee without exploitation of people or planet. They
produce a wonderful redbush tea 'lookalike' which is great for those
trying to reduce their tea consumption. Clipper teas are available
from most major supermarkets and health food stores.

Doves Farm Foods Ltd

Salisbury Road, Hungerford, Berkshire RG17 0RF.
Tel: 01488 684880, www.dovesfarm.co.uk

An ever increasing range of organic products from cereals, home baking flours and cookies to snack bars and bread. Selected items available from all major supermarkets and health food stores.

Breakfast cereals
Snack bars
Gluten free biscuits
Speciality flour

Evernat

Brewhurst Health Food Supplies Ltd, Abbot Close, Oyster Lane, Byfleet, Surrey KT13 7JP.
Tel: 01932 354211, email: k-shaw@brewhurst.com,
www.brewhurst.com

Providing delicious organic products, from cereals and snack bars to prepared frozen meals and condiments.

Almond and hazelnut milk
Soya milk
Dried skimmed milk powder
Dried soya milk powder
Mayonnaise
Crunchy oat cereal
Cereal snack bars

Gluten Free Foods Ltd

Unit 270 Centennial Park, Centennial Avenue, Elstree, Hertfordshire WD6 3SS.
Tel: 0208 9534444, email: ellis@glutenfree-foods.co.uk,
www.glutenfree-foods.co.uk

Gluten Free Foods Ltd supply a range of over 40 wheat free and gluten free products under their Barkat and Glutano brands. Most products are also free of lactose, egg, soya and yeast.

Barkat white and brown rice bread
Glutano gluten free bread, rolls
Gluten free flour and bread mixes

Pasta
Cakes, biscuits

Haldane Foods

Howard Way, Newport Pagnell, Buckinghamshire MK16 9PY.
Tel: 01908 211311, www.haldanefoods.co.uk

Haldane Foods are experts in meat-free and non-dairy foods, selling
products under the brand names of Granose and Realeat.

Realeat meat replacement ready made meals
Granose Soya milk
Granose Soya milk shakes
Organic range of snack pot meals and prepared vegetarian meals

Heinz

HJ Heinz Co, Stockley Park, Uxbridge, Middlesex UB11 1HZ.
Tel: 0208 5737757, www.heinz.co.uk

Heinz are moving into the organic market, with the introduction of
organic varieties of most their best selling products. Organic baked
beans, tomato ketchup and now they have two new soya milk
products, original organic and vanilla.

Baked beans
Tinned spaghetti
Tomato ketchup
Organic soya milk
Vanilla soya milk

Innocent Drinks

Fruit Towers, 3 Goldhawk Estate, Brackenbury Road, London W6
0BA.
Tel: 0208 6003939, email: daisy@innocentdrinks.co.uk,
www.innocentdrinks.co.uk

Innocent use only fresh ingredients for their smoothies and thickies,
with no concentrated juices, colourings or flavourings. Each drink
contains the recommended daily allowance of fresh fruit. Available

from Sainsburys and Waitrose, and most health food stores.
Fruit smoothies (pure fruit pulp)
Thickies (yogurt and fruit)
Veggies (vegetable juice)

Jordan's

W Jordan (Cereals) Ltd, Holme Mills, Biggleswade, Bedfordshire
SG18 9JY.
Tel: 01767 318222, www.jordancereals.co.uk

Pioneers in developing natural foods, leading the market in organic
cereals and bars. All products in the Jordan's range use conservation
grade cereals which respects the environment as well as our health.
Most products are available in all major supermarkets and health
food stores.

Oat crunchy cereals
Frusli cereal bars
Savoury snacks

Joubère

Coastal Trading Ltf, 6 & 7 Dukes Road, London W3 0SL.
Tel: 020 8992 6851, email: replies@joubere.co.uk

Joubère are the UK market leaders in the manufacture of high
quality chilled fresh stock, soup, gravy and dairy desserts. Most
products are organic. Available from Sainsburys and Waitrose and
most some major health food stores.

Fresh custard
Rice pudding with fruit coulis
Pannacotta with wild blueberry
Porridge
Noodles
Fresh chicken/vegetable stock

Lawncourt Harvest

Aldeburgh Road, Friston, Suffolk IP17 1NP.
Tel: 01728 689197, www.munchyseeds.com

Mixed dry roasted seeds in a dash of savoury sauce, suitable for gluten and dairy free diets. Ideal to liven up a salad or as a wholesome snack at any time of the day. Great for adding to homemade bread and veggie stir-fries. A great source of omega-6 essential fatty acids.

Original – sunflower seeds, sesame seeds, soya beans, sea salt, koji
Pumpkin – with the addition of pumpkin seeds

LoSalt

Klinge Foods Ltd, 1 Bessemer Drive, Kelvin Industrial Estate, East Kilbride, Glasgow G75 0QX.
Tel: 01355 238464, email: enquiries@losalt.com

Manufacturers of reduce sodium salt alternative, which is recommended for anyone who needs to reduce their sodium intake. A reduced sodium diet is particularly important for those with fluid retention, and more seriously high blood pressure. LoSalt can be utilised in the same way as conventional salt, and is available from all major supermarkets.

Lyme Regis Foods

Unit D, Station Road Industrial Estate, Liphook, Hampshire GU30 7DR.
Tel: 01428 722900, email: info@lymeregisfoods.com,
www.lymeregisfoods.com

Manufacturers of a range of healthy snack foods, both organic and non-organic. All are made from natural ingredients and are suitable for vegetarians, and free from hydrogenated fat. Some products in the range are dairy, wheat and gluten free. Available from most health food stores.

Fruit and cereal bars
Flapjacks
Marzipan bars

Meridian Foods

Unit 13, WDA Advance Factories, Corwen, Denbighshire LL21 9RJ.
Tel: 01490 413151, email: lrowlands@meridianfoods.co.uk,
www.meridianfoods.co.uk

Ever expanding its range, Meridian endeavours to produce high
quality organic products at affordable prices. Sample some delicious
foods, including pasta sauces, fruit spreads, peanut butter and
condiments. Available from major supermarkets and health food
stores.

Pure fruit spread
Salad dressings
Marinades
Fruit juice concentrates
Pasta sauce
Pasta

Nairn's Oatcakes

90 Peffermill Road, Edinburgh, Mid Lothian EH16 5UU.
Tel: 0131 6207000, email: walter@simmersofedinburgh.co.uk,
www.simmers-nairn's.co.uk

Nairn's is the leading producer of oatcakes. The range includes
products that are organic, wheat free, sugar free and high in fibre.
Available from all supermarkets and health food stores.

Oatcakes – several varieties

Nature's Path

7453 Progress Way, Delta, BC, V4G 1E8, Canada.
Tel: (604) 9400505, email: cereal@naturespath.bc.ca,
www.naturespath.com

Organic multigrain and, wheat free and gluten free cereals. Available
from selected supermarkets and most health food stores.

Cornflakes
Heritage Muesli

Multigrain Flakes
Millet Rice
Blueberry almond muesli
Heritage O's
Mesa Sunrise

Orgran

Community Foods Ltd, Micross, Brent Terrace, London NW2 1LT.
Tel: 020 82082966, colin.winter@communityfoods.co.uk,
www.communityfoods.co.uk

The Orgran range caters for people with specific food sensitivity problems free from gluten, wheat and dairy. Available from some Sainsburys and Waitrose stores, and most health food stores.

Rice cakes
Corn cakes
Pasta – spaghetti, lasagne, macaroni
Bread mixes
Falafel mix

Pete & Johnny's Plc

15 Lots Road, Chelsea Wharf, London SW10 0QT.
Tel: 0207 3520276, email: ellen@p-j.co.uk, www.p-j.co.uk

Pete and Johnny's Smoothies contain only the finest fresh fruit to make a thick, juicy pulp, with nothing added and nothing taken away. Available from most major supermarkets and health food stores.

100 per cent pure fruit smoothies

Plamil Foods

Plamil House, Bowles Well Gardens, Folkestone, Kent CT19 6PQ.
Tel: 01303 850588, email: contactus@plamilfoods.co.uk,
www.plamilfoods.co.uk

Plamil is extending its organic range of products to feature dairy free organic chocolate, mayonnaise and other condiments.

Soya milk – sweetened and unsweetened
Mayonnaise – gluten, dairy, egg free
Organic dairy free chocolate bars
Carob

Princess

Royal Liver Building, Pier Head, Liverpool L3 1NX.
Tel: 0151 236 9282

Princess have a range of tasty tinned fish, including mackerel and sardines in tomato sauce or olive oil. Oily fish is a particularly good source of essential fatty acids, and a good non-dairy source of calcium, necessary for healthy bones. All products in the Princess range are available from supermarkets.

Provamel

Alpro UK Ltd, Altendiez Way, Latimer Business Park, Burton Latimer, Northamptonshire NN15 5YZ.
Tel: 01536 720605

A range of soya based products including Soya Fruity, an organic soya juice drink and yofu yogurt in a range of flavours. Provamel are just launching their latest addition, fresh chilled soya milk. The full range is available from most major supermarkets and health food stores.

Rachel's Dairy

Leigh Manor, Minsterley, Shropshire SY5 0EX.
Tel: 01743 891990, d.stacey@dial.pipex.com, www.rachelsorganic.co.uk

Producers of delicious top quality organic dairy products made in Wales to the highest standards. Made to unique family recipes and using only fresh organic liquid milk. Rachel's products do not contain any artificial thickeners, flavours or colours.

Natural yogurt – wholemilk and semi-skimmed
Fruit yoghurts
Greek yogurt
Natural yogurt with maple syrup

Natural yogurt with honey
Crème fraîche

The Village Bakery

The Village Bakery, Melmerby, Penrith, Cumbria CA10 1HE.
Tel: 01768 881515, email: info@village-bakery.com,
www.village-bakery.com

The Village Bakery is the leading British organic bakery brand.
Using traditional methods it has won numerous awards for its
innovative breads, cakes, biscuits and Christmas specialities. It
supplies nationwide to natural food shops, food halls, caterers and
multiples.

Gluten free bread
Wheat free bread
French bread
Wholemeal bread
Wheat free cakes and biscuits

Tropical Wholefoods

7 Stradella Road, Herne Hill, London SE24 9HN.
Tel: 0207 7370444, email: tropicalwf@aol.com,
www.tropicalwholefoods.com

Sun dried organic and natural tropical fruits from all over the world,
bursting with flavour. Available from most health food stores.

Dried mango, papaya, banana
Muesli
Tropical fruit bars
Banana and oat bars

Tropicana

126-128 Cromwell Road, London SW7 4ET.
Tel: 020 7370 5675

Tropicana produces a range of freshly squeezed fruit juices, ranging
from orange to apple and cranberry. All products are naturally rich

in vitamin C, but they have a variety of orange juice with added calcium which is ideal for people with busy lifestyles who may have a higher requirement for this important mineral, but may not eat fish and dairy products (which are naturally rich in calcium) on a daily basis. Tropicana is widely available from all supermarkets.

Twinings Teas

R Twining & Co Ltd, South Way, Andover, Hampshire SP10 5AQ.
Tel: 01264 334477

Twinings offer an extensive range of herbal and fruit infusions, including the new exotic blends, plus the award winning range of organic infusions and speciality teas. Available from all supermarkets and health food stores.

Whole Earth

2 Valentine Place, London SE1 8QH.
Tel: 0207 6335900, email: clunyb@wholeearthfoods.co.uk,
www.wholeearthfoods.com

The pioneering organic food company have been dedicated to healthy eating since 1967. They make a delicious range of organic foods including breakfast cereals, peanut butter and soft drinks. All Whole Earth products are certified by the Soil Association. Most products available from all major supermarkets and health food stores.

Peanut butter
Fruit spread
Condiments
Cereals
Soft drinks
NoCaf
Baked beans

Women's Nutritional Advisory Service (WNAS)

PO Box 268, Lewes, East Sussex BN7 1QN.
Tel: 01273 487366, Fax: 01273 487576, Mail Order Service: 0845 6012765, email: wnas@wnas.org.uk, www.wnas.org.uk

Yeo Valley

Yeo Valley Organic Co Ltd, Cannington, Somerset TA5 2ND.
Tel: 01278 652243

Specialising in organic dairy products and chilled goods. Available
from all major supermarkets and health food stores.
Bio natural and fruit yoghurts
Crème fraîche
Cream
Fruit compôte

APPENDIX

Useful addresses

AAA (Action Against Allergy)
PO Box 278
Twickenham TW1 4QQ
Tel: 0208 892 2711

ACCEPT Clinic
724 Fulham Road
London SW6 5SE
Tel: 0207 371 7477

Al-Anon Family Groups
61 Great Dover Street
London SE1 4YF
Tel: 0207 403 0888

Albany Trust Counselling
St Paul's Centre
Rossmore Road
London NW1 6NJ
Tel: 0208 767 1827

Alcohol Concern
Waterbridge House
32-36 Loman Street
London SE1 0EE
Tel: 0207 928 7377

Alcohol Counselling Prevention
Services
34 Electric Lane
London SW9 8JT
Tel: 0207 737 3579

Alcoholics Anonymous (AA)
General Services Office
PO Box 1
Stonebow House
York YO1 7NJ
Tel: 0845 7697555

Allan Sweeney International Reiki and
Healing Training Centre
10 Beech Houses
Royal Crescent
Margate
Kent CT9 5AL
Tel: 01843 230377
www.reiki-healing.com

Allergycare
Health Screening Ltd
1 Church Square
Taunton
Somerset TA1 1SA
Tel: 01823 325023

Anorexia and Bulimia Care
PO Box 30
Ormskirk
Lancashire L39 5JR
Tel: 01695 422479

ASH (Action on Smoking and Health)
102 Clifton Street
London EC2A 4HW
Tel: 0207 840 8300

British Diabetic Association
10 Queen Anne Street
London W1G 9LH
Tel: 0207 323 1531

British Dyslexia Association
98 London Road
Reading
Berks RG1 5AU
Tel: 0118 966 2677

British Epilepsy Association
New Anstey House
Gateway Drive
Yeadon
Leeds LS19 7XY
Tel: 0113 210 8800

British Migraine Association
178A High Road
West Byfleet
Surrey KT14 7ED
Tel: 01932 352468

British Pregnancy Advisory Service
Austy Manor
Wootton Wawen
Solihull
West Midlands B95 6BX
Tel: 01564 793225

British School of Osteopathy
Administration and Clinics
275 Borough High Street
London SE1 1JE
Tel: 0207 930 9254

British Society for Allergy and
Clinical Immunology
66 Western Park
Thames Ditton
Surrey KT7 0HL
Tel: 0208 398 9240

British Society for Haematology
2 Carlton House Terrace
London SW1Y 5AF
Tel: 0208 643 7305

British Society of Allergy and
Environmental Medicine
PO Box 7
Knighton RD7 1WT
Tel: 01703 812124

British Wheel of Yoga
1 Hamilton Place
Boston Road
Sleaford
Lincolnshire NG34 7ES
Tel: 01529 306851

Coeliac Society
PO Box 220
High Wycombe
Buckinghamshire HP11 2HY
Tel: 01494 437278

College of Health
St Margaret's House
21 Old Ford Road
London E2 9PL
Tel: 0208 983 1225

Daisy Chain Network
PO Box 392
High Wycombe
Buckinghamshire HP27 0AE
www.daisychain.org.uk

Depression Alliance
35 Westminster Bridge Road
London SE1 7JP
Tel: 0207 633 0557

Drugaid
16 Clive Street
Caerphilly CF83 1GE
Tel: 02920 881000

Eating Disorders Association
1st Floor
Wensum House
103 Prince of Wales Road
Norwich
NR1 1DW
01603 621414

Friends of the Earth Ltd
26-28 Underwood Street
London N1 7JQ
Tel: 0207 490 1555

General Council and Register of
Naturopaths
Goswell House
Street
Somerset BA16 0JG
Tel: 01458 840072

London Food Commission
3rd Floor
5-11 Worship Street
London EC21 2BH
Tel: 0207 7837 2250

Migraine Trust
45 Great Ormond Street
London WC1N 3HZ
Tel: 0207 831 4818

MIND
15-19 Broadway
Stratford
London WC1N 4BO
Tel: 0208 519 2122

National Abortion Campaign
The Print House
18 Ashwin Street
London E8 3DL
Tel: 0207 923 4976

National Aids Helpline: 0800 567123

National Asthma Campaign
Providence House
Providence Place
London N1 0NT
Tel: 0207 226 2260

National Council for One-Parent
Families
255 Kentish Town Road
London NW5 2LX
Tel: 0800 018 5026

National Eczema Society
163 Eversholt Street
London NW1 1BU
Tel: 0870 241 3604

National Endometriosis Society
Suite 50
Westminster Palace Gardens
1-7 Artillery Row
London SW1R 1RL
Tel: 0207 222 2776

British Pregnancy Advisory Service
26 Bedford Square
London WC1B 3HH
Tel: 0207 637 8962
QUIT
Victory House
170 Tottenham Court Road
London W1P 0HA
Tel: 0207 487 3000

Rape Crisis Centre
PO Box 69
London WC1X 9NJ
Emergency Tel: 0207 837 1600
(6–10pm and weekends only)

Raynaud's and Scleroderma
Association
112 Crewe Road
Alsager
Cheshire ST7 2JA
Tel: 01270 872776

Terence Higgins Trust
52-54 Grays Inn Road
London WC1X 8JU
Tel: 0207 831 0330
Helpline: 0207 242 1010

Tranx (UK) Ltd
National Tranquilliser Advice
Centre
25a Masons Avenue
Wealdstone
Harrow
Middlesex
HA3 5AH
Tel: 020 8427 2065 (client line);
020 8427 2827 (24hr answering
service)

Vegan Society
Donald Watson House
7 Battle Road
St Leonards on Sea
East Sussex TN3Y 7AA
Tel: 01424 427393

Vegetarian Society
Parkdale
Dunham Road
Altrincham
Cheshire WA14 4QG
Tel: 0161 928 0793

Verity
52-42 Featherstone Street
London EC1Y 8RT
Tel: 020 7251 9009
www.verity-pcos.org.uk

References

STANDARD REFERENCES:

1. Prescription for Nutritional Healing – 2nd edition, Balch, J, Balch, P, Avery, 1997
2. Textbook of Nutritional Medicine, Werbach, M, Moss, J, Third Line Press, 1999
3. Textbook of Natural Medicine – Volume 1 & 2, Pizzorno, J, Murray, M, Churchill Livingstone, 1999
4. Environmental Medicine in Clinical Practice, Anthony, H et al, BSAENM Publications, 1997
5. Encyclopedia of Complementary Medicine – The definitive guide to the best
6. Treatment options for 200 health problems, Woodham, A and Peters Dr D,
7. Dorling Kindersely, 1997
8. Human Nutrition And Dietetics, by R. Passmore & M.A. Eastwood, Eighth Edition, published by Churchill Livingstone, Edinburgh 1986.
9. Nutritional Medicine, by Dr Stephen Davies & Dr Alan Stewart, published by Pan Books, London 1987

ABDOMINAL WIND:

1. Maxton, D.G., Martin, D.F., Whorwell, P.J., Godfrey, M. Abdominal distension in female patients with irritable bowel syndrome; exploration of possible mechanisms. Gut.1991;32:62-64.
2. Cummings, J.H. Fermentation in the human large intestine: evidence and implications for health. The Lancet. 1983;1:1206-1209.
3. Hunter, J.O. Food allergy - or enterometabolic disorder? The Lancet. 1991;2:495-496.
4. Calloway, S.P. , Fonagy, P. Aerophagia and irritable bowel syndrome. The Lancet. 1985;2:1368.
5. Levitt, M.D., Lasser, R.N., Schwartz, J.S., Bond, J.H. Studies of a flatulent patient. The New England Journal of Medicine. 1976;295:260-262.

6. Editorial. The colon, the rumen, and d-lactic acidosis. The Lancet. 1990;336:599-600.
7. Trotman, I.F., Price, C.C. Bloated irritable bowel syndrome defined by dynamic 99m Tc Bran Scan. The Lancet. 1986;2:364-366.
8. Christi, S.U. Gibson, G.R., Cummmings, J.H. Role of dietary sulphate in the regulation of methanogenesis in the human large intestine. Gut.1992;33:1234-1238.

ACNE
Standard references

ACNE ROSACIA
Standard references

AGORAPHOBIA
1. Burns, L.E. Thorpe, G.L. Fears and Clinical Phobias: Epidemiological Aspects and The National Survey of Agoraphobics. Journal of International Medical Research. Vol 5(1) 1977.

ANAEMIA
1. Lucas , C.A., Logan, E.C.N. & Logan, R.A..Audit of the Investigation and Outcome of Iron Deficiency anaemia in one health district. Journal of the Royal College of Physicians of London. 1996; 33-3

ANXIETY
Standard references plus
1. Durham R, Allan T. Psychological treatment of generalised anxiety disorder: a review of the clinical significance of results in outcome studies since 980. Br J Psychol 1993; 163: 19-26

BREAST PROBLEMS
1. Boyle, C.A. et al. Caffeine Consumption and Fibrocystic Breast Disease: A Case Control Epidemiologic Study. JNCI. 72:1015-1019, 1984
2. London, R.S. et al. The Effect of Alpha-Toocopherol on

Premenstrual Sympomatology: A Double-Blind Study 2. Endocrine correlates. Journal of American College of Nutrition. 3:351-356. 1884

3. Boyd E.M.F et al. The effect of a low-fat, high complex-carbohydrate diet -on symptoms of cyclical mastopathy. The Lancet. 2:128-132. 1988.
4. Mansel RE, Breast Pain "ABC of Breast Diseases". BMJ 1994; 309: 866-868
5. Gateley CA, et Al Drug treatments for mastalgia: 17 years' experience in the Cardiff mastalgia clinic. Journal of the Royal Society of Medicien 1992; 85:12-15
6. Hughes LE et al, Benign Disorders and Diseases of the Breast. 1989, Bailliere Tindll, London.

CONSTIPATION

1. Editorial. Constipation in young women. The Lancet.1986;1:778-779.
2. Turnbull, G.K., Lennard-Jones, J.E., Bartram, C.I. Failure of rectal expulsion as a cause of constipation: why fibre and laxatives sometimes fail. The Lancet. 1986;1767-769.
3. Preston, D.M., Lennard-Jones, J.E. Severe chronic constipation of young women: 'idiopathic slow transit constipation'. Gut.1986;27:41-48.
4. Cann, P.A., Read, N.W., Holdsworth, C.D. What is the benefit of wheat bran in patients with irritable bowel syndrome? Gut.1984;25:168-173.
5. Alun Jones, V., McLaughlan, P., Shorthouse, M., Workman, E., Hunter, J.O. Food intolerance: a major factor in the pathogenesis of irritable bowel syndrome. The Lancet. 1982;2:1115-1117.
6. Taylor, R. Management of constipation. British Medical Journal 1990;300:1065-1067.
7. Hojgaard, L., Arffman, S., Jorgensen, M., Kragg, E. Tea consumption a cause of constipation. British Medical Journal 1981;282:864.

DEPRESSION

1. Riley, D.M., Watt, D.C., 'Hypercalcemia in the Etiology of

Puerperal Psychosis', Society of Biological Psychiatry, 1985; 20: 479-488.

2. Dostalova, L., 'Vitamin status during puerperium and lactation', *Annals of Nutrition and Metabolism* (1984) 28 (6) 385-408 [En 27 ref] Dep. Vitamin and Nutrition Research, F. Hoffmann-La Roche & Co Ltd, CH-4002, Basle, Switzerland.

3. Watson, J.P., Elliott, S.A., Rugg, A.J., Brough, D.I., 'Psychiatric Disorder in Pregnancy and the First Postnatal Year', *British Journal of Psychiatry*, 1984: 144; 453-462.

DERMATITIS

1. Hunter J.A.A. and Herd R.M. Recent advances in atopic dermatitis. Quarterly Journal of Medicine. 1994;87:323-327.

DIABETES

1. McNair et. al. Hypomagnesemia: a risk factor in diabetic retinopathy. *Diabetes,* 1978;27:1075-1077.

2. Moles, K.W., & McMullen, J.K., 'Insulin resistance and hypomagnesaemia, case report', *British Medical Journal,* 1982;285:262.

3. Coelingh Bennink, H.J.T., & Schreurs, W.H.P., 'Improvement of oral glucose tolerance in gestational diabetes by pyridoxine', *British Medical Journal,* 1975;3;13-15.

DIARRHOEA

1. Report by the Royal College of Physicians. 1984: Food Allergy and Intolerance.

2. Cooper, B.T. , Holmes, G.K.T., Ferguson, R.A., Thompson, R.N.A., Cooke, W.T. Gluten-sensitive diarrhoea without evidence of coeliac disease. Gastroenterology. 1980;79:801-806.

3. Arnason, J.A., Gudjonsson, H., Freysodottir, J., Jonsdottir, I., Valdimarsson, H. Do adults with high gliadin antibody concentrations have subclinical gluten intolerance? Gut. 1992;33:194-197.

4. Editorial. Milk fat, diarrhoea and the ileal brake. The Lancet.1986;2:658.

5. Editorial. Hastening Gut Transit. The LANCET. L990;2:974.

6. Merliss, R.R., Hofman, A. Steatorrhoea following the use of antibiotics. The New England Journal of Medicine. l95l;245:328-330.
7. Bennett, J.R. Progress Report: Smoking and the gastrointestinal tract. Gut. l972;13:658-665.

EATING DISORDERS

1. Lacey, J.H., 'Bulimia nervosa, binge eating and psychogenic vomiting: a controlled treatment study and long-term outcome', *British Medical Journal*, 1993;286:1609-1613.

ECZEMA

1. Sloper K.S., Wadsworth J. and Brostoff J. Children with atopic eczema. 1: Clinical response to food elimination and subsequent double-blind food challenge. Quarterly Journal of medicine. 1991;80:677-693.
2. Morse P.F. et al. Meta-analysis of placebo-controlled studies of the efficacy of Epogam in the treatment of atopic eczema. Relationship between essential fatty acid changes and clinical response. British Journal of Dermatology. 1989;121:75-90.
3. Turner M.A., Devlin J. and David T.J. Holidays and atopic eczema. Archives of Disease in Childhood. 1991;66:212-21.

ENDOMETRIOSIS

Standard references plus:
1. Endometriosis – a key to healing through nutrition, Mills, D, Vernon, M, Element, 1999
2. Natural Treatment of Fibroid Tumours and Endometriosis – effective natural solutions for relieving heavy bleeding, cramps and infertility that accompany these common female problems, Susan M. Lark, M.DE., Keats Publishing

FATIGUE

1. Jenkins, R., and Mowbray, W. (eds), *Post-Viral Fatigue Syndrome*, John Wiley & Sons, Chichester, UK, 1990.
2. Behan, P., Goldberg, G. and Mowbray, J.F., 'Post-viral fatigue syndrome', *British Medical Bulletin*, 47, No 4, 1991.
3. Manu, P., Lane, T.J. and Matthews, D.A., 'The frequency of

chronic fatigue syndrome in patients with persistent fatigue',
Annals of International Medicine, 1988; 109: 554

FIBROIDS

Standard references plus:

1. Natural Treatment of Fibroid Tumours and Endometriosis –
   effective natural solutions for relieving heavy bleeding, cramps
   and infertility that accompany these common female problems,
   Susan M. Lark, M.DE., Keats Publishing

FOOD CRAVING

Standard references plus

1. Beat Sugar Craving by Maryon Stewart. Published by
   Vermilion, 1992.

GASTROENTEROLOGICAL PROBLEMS

1. Lennard Jones, L.E., 'Nutrition and Crohn's Disease', *Annals of
   the Royal College of Surgeons of England,* 1990;72:152-4.
2. Hawthorne, A.B., 'Treatment of ulcerative colitis with fish oil
   supplementation: a prospective 12-month randomised
   controlled trial'. *Gut,* 1992;33:922-928
3. Pearson, D.J., Stones, N.A., Bentley, S.J. & Reid, H.,
   'Protocolitis induced by salicylate and associated with asthma
   and recurrent nasal polyps', *British Medical Journal,*
   1983;287:1675.
4. Hill, S.M., & Mills, P.J., 'Colitis caused by food allergy in
   infants', *Archives of Diseases in Childhood,* 1990; 65:132-40.
5. Wright, R., & Truelove, S.C., 'A controlled therapeutic trial of
   various diets in ulcerative colitis', *British Medical Journal,*
   1965;2:138-41.
6. Pitcher, M.C.L., Beatty, E.R. & Cummings, J.H., 'Salicylates
   inhibit bacterial sulphide production within the colonic
   lumen', Gut, 1995;37 (supp12):A15.

HAIR LOSS

Standard references

HALITOSIS

1. Kerr, D.A., Major M. Ash, Jr., Oral Pathology, Lea & Febiger, sixth edition, Philadelphia, 1992.

IBS

1. Connell A.M., Hilton C., Irvine G. et al, 'Variation of bowel habit in two population samples', *British Medical Journal* 1965;2:1095-1099
2. Drossman D.A., Sandler R.S., McKee D.C., Lovitz A.J., *Bowel patterns among subjects not seeking health care*, *Gastroenterology* 1982;83:529-34.
3. Heaton K.W., O'Donnell L.J.D., Braddon F.E.M., Mountford R.A., Hughes A.O., Cripps P.J., *Gastroenterology* 1992; 102:1962-1967.
4. Danivat D., Tankeyoon M., Sritratanaban A., 'Prevalence of irritable bowel syndrome in a non-Western population', *British Medical Journal*. 1988;296:17105
5. Jones R., Lydeard S., 'Irritable bowel syndrome in the general population', *British Medical Journal*, 1992;304:87-90
6. Isgar B., Harman M., Kaye M.D., Whorwell P.J., 'Symptoms of irritable bowel syndrome in ulcerative colitis in remission', *Gut*. 1983;24:190-192
7. Whitehead, W.E., et al, Effects of stressful life events on bowel symptoms:
8. subjects with irritable bowel syndrome compared with subjects without bowel dysfunction. Gut. 1992; 33:825-30.
9. Thompson, W.G., `Irritable bowel syndrome: pathogenesis and management. The Lancet. 1993; 341:1569-72.
10. No More IBS!, Maryon Stewart & Dr Alan Stewart, Vermilion, 1999

INSOMNIA

Standard references plus

1. Coyle, K., Watts F.N., *The factorial structure of sleep dissatisfaction*. Behave Res Ther 1991; 29:315-20
2. Ford, D.E., Kamerow, D.B. *Epidemiological study of sleep disturbances and psychiatric disturbances.* JAMA 1989; 262:1479-84

3. *The Medical Management of Insomnia In General Practice*, edited by Malcolm Lader, Royal Society of Medicine, London, 1992

MIGRAINE

7. Hannington, E., Jones, R.J. *et al*, 'Migraine: a platelet disorder', *The Lancet*, ii (981), 720-23.
8. Egger, J., Carter, C.M. *et al*, 'Is migraine a food allergy? A double-blind controlled trial of oligoantigenic diet treatment', *The Lancet*, ii (1983), 865-9.
9. Monro, J., Carini, C., Brostoff, J., 'Migraine is a food-allergic disease', *The Lancet* ii (1984), 719-21.
10. Grant, E., 'Food allergies in migraine', *The Lancet*, I (1979), 966-9.
11. Lance, J.W., 'Treatment of Migraine', *The Lancet*, 1992; 339:1207-1209.
12. Murphy, J.J., Heptinstall, S., Mitchell, J.R.A., 'Randomised double-blind placebo-controlled trial of feverfew in migraine prevention', *The Lancet*, 1988; 189.
13. Lockett, D-MC, Campbell, J.F., 'The effects of aerobic exercise on migraine', *Headache*, 1992; 32:
14. 50-54.
15. Iversen, H.K., Nielsen, T.H., Olesen, J., Tfelt-Hansen, P., 'Arterial responses during migraine headaches', The Lancet, 1990; 336: 837-39.
16. Epstein, M.T., Hockaday, J.M., Hockaday, T.D.R., 'Migraine and reproductive hormones throughout the menstrual cycle', The Lancet, 1975; 543-548.
17. Buring, J.E., Peto, R., Hennekens, C.H., 'Low-dose Aspirin for Migraine Prophylaxis', JAMA, 1990: 264: 1711-1713.
18. Kew, J., McKeran, R., 'Prophylactic treatment of migraine', Maternal and Child Health, 1991: 46-51.
19. Egger, J., 'Psychoneurological aspects of food allergy', European Journal of Clinical Nutrition, 1991: 45 (Suppl. 1), 35-45.

MOUTH DISORDERS

1. Editorial, 'Apthous ulceration', *Journal of the Royal Society of Medicine*, 1994; 77: 1-3.
2. Lamey, P.J., Hammond, A., Allam, B.F., McIntosh, W.B., '

Vitamin status of patients with burning mouth syndrome and the response to replacement therapy', *British Dental Journal*, 1986; 160: 81.

3. Strean, L.P., Bell, F.T., Gilfillan, E.W., Emerson, G.A., Howe, E.E., 'The importance of pyridoxine in the suppression of dental caries in school children and hamsters', *New York State Dental Journal*, 1958; 24: 133.

4. Ferguson, M.M., 'Disorders of the mouth in clinical practice', *Medicine in Practice*, 1982; Vol 1: No. 9: 243-7.

NAIL PROBLEMS
Standard references

OVARIAN CYSTS
Standard references

PAINFUL OVULATION
Standard references

PELVIC INFLAMMATORY DISEASE
Standard references

POLYCYSTIC OVARIES

1. McCluskey, S.E., Lacey, J.H., Pearce, J.M., 'Binge-eating and polycystic ovaries', *The Lancet*, 1992: 340; 723.

2. Kiddy, D.S., Hamilton-Fairley, D., Bush, A., Short, F., Anyaoku, V., Reed, M.J., Franks, S., 'Improvements in endocrine and ovarian function during dietary treatment of obese women with polycystic ovary syndrome', *Clinical Endrocrinology*, 1992: 36; 105-111.

3. Macaulay, J.H., Bond, K., Steet, P.J., 'Epidural analgesia in labor and fetal hyperthermia', *Obstetrics and Gynaecology*, 1992; 80: 665-9.

4. Polson, D.W., Adams, J., Wadsworth, J., Franks, S., 'Polycystic ovaries - a common finding in normal women', *The Lancet*, 1988:870.

PRECONCEPTION

1. Barker, D.J.P., *Mothers, Babies, and Disease in Later Life*, British Medical Journal, Publishing Group, 1994

2. Wynn, M., Wynn, A., 'New thoughts on maternal nutrition', The Caroline Walker Lecture 1993,

3. Widdowson, E.M., McCance, R.A., 'A review: new thoughts on growth', *Paediatric Research*, 1975; 9: 154-6.

4. Barker, D.J.P. *et al*, 'Weight in infancy and death from ischaemic heart disease', *The Lancet*,1989; ii: 577-80.

5. Osmond, C., Barker, D.J.P. *et al*, 'Early growth and death from cardiovascular disease in women', *British Medical Journal*, 1993; 307: 1519-24.

PREGNANCY

1. Barker, D.J.P., *Mothers, Babies and Disease in Later Life*, British *Medical Journal*, Publishing Group , 1994.

2. *Vitamin A and pregnancy*, Chief Medical Officer, Department of Health letters to all doctors, October 1990 and November 1993.

3. 'Routine iron supplements in pregnancy are unnecessary', *British National Formulary*, April 1994.

4. Czeizel, A.E., 'Periconceptional multivitamin supplementation in prevention of congenital abnormalities', *Maternal and Child Health*, December 1994; 381-4.

5. Kirke, P.N., Molloy, A.M., Daly, L.E. *et al*, 'Maternal plasma folate and vitamin B12 are independent risk factors for neural tube defects', *Quarterly Journal of Medicine*, 1993; 86: 703-8.

6. Laroque, B. *et al*, 'Effects on birth weight of alcohol and caffeine consumption during pregnancy', *American Journal of Epidemiology*, 1993; 137; (9): 941-50.

7. Spohr, H.L. *et al*, 'Prenatal alcohol exposure and long-term development consequences', *The Lancet*, 1993; 341: 907-10.

8. Dolan-Mullen, P. *et al*, 'A meta-analysis of randomized trials of prenatal smoking cessation interventions', *American Journal of Obstetrics and Gynaecology*, 1994; 1328-34.

9. Czeizel, A.E. *et al*, 'Smoking during pregnancy and congenital limb deficiency', *British Medical Journal*, 1994; 308: 1473-6.

PREMENSTRUAL SYNDROME

1. Green R., Dalton K. The premenstrual Syndrome. British Medical Journal, May 9 1953. P1007-1014.
2. Morton J.H., Additon H., Addison R.G., Hunt L., Sullivan J.J. A clinical study of Premenstrual Tension. A.M.J. Obstet. Gynecol. 55:1182-1191. 1953.
3. Sherwood R.A., Rocks, B.F., Stewart A., Saxton R.S. Magnesium in the Pre-Menstrual Syndrome. Ann. Clin. Biochem. 23:667-670. 1986.
4. Ashton C.H. Caffeine and Health. The British medical Journal. 295:1293-4. 1987.
5. Chakmakjian Z,H., Higgins C.E., Abraham G.E. The Effect of a Nutritional Supplement, Optivite, for Women with Pre-Menstrual Tension Syndromes: 2. The effect of Symtomatology, using a Double-Blind Cross-Over Design. The Journal of Applied Nutrition. 37:1-11. 1986.
6. No More PMS!, Stewart, M & Stewart, Dr Alan, Vermilion, 1997

PSORIASIS

1. Menter A. and Barker J.N.W.N. Psoriasis in practice. The Lancet. 1991;338:231-234.
2. Maurice P.D.L., Allen B.R., Barkley A.S.J., Cockbill S.R., Stammers J. and Bather P.C. The effects of dietary supplementation with fish oil in patients with psoriasis. British Journal of Dermatology. 1987;117:599-606.
3. Michaelsson G., Gerden B., Ottosson M. et al. Patients with psoriasis often have increased serum levels of IgA antibodies to gliadin. British Journal of Dermatology. 1993;129:667-673.
4. Rowland Payne C.M.E. Psoriatic science. British Medical Journal. 1987;295:1158-y

VAGINAL PROBLEMS

Standard references plus

1. Witkins SS, Jeremias J Ledger WJ. Recurrent vaginitis as a result of sexual transmission of IgE antibodies. Am J Obstet Gynecol 1988; 159:32-36

Recommended reading

GENERAL

The Natural Health Bible, M Stewart & Dr A Stewart (Vermilion)
Maryon Stewart's Zest for Life Plan, M Stewart (Headline)
Better Health through Natural Healing, R Trattler (Thorsons)
Optimal Wellness, Ralph Golan (Ballantine Books)
Feel Fabulous Forever, J Fairley & S Stacey (Kyle Cathie)
Perfect Skin, A Cochrane (Piatkus)
The Beauty Bible, J Fairley & S Stacey (Kyle Cathie)
MSM The Natural Pain Relief, Deborah Mitchell (Wholecare)
Fats that Heal Fats the Kill, Udo Erasmus (Alive Books)
Why I can't remember, Pavel Yutsis & Lynda Toth (Avery
    Publishing)
Mental Health the Nutrition Connection, Patrick Holford (Piatkus)
Food for Fitness, Amanda Bean (A & C Black)
Conquering Cystitis, Dr Patrick Kingsley (Ebury Press)

FOOD

The New Foods Guide, John Elkington & Julia Hailes (Gollancz
    Publishing)
The Food Bible, Judith Wills (Quadrille Publishing Ltd)
Foods that Harm Foods that Heal (Reader's Digest)
Beat Sugar Craving, M Stewart (Vermilion)
The Allergy Diet, Elizabeth Workman, SRD, Dr John Hunter and
    Dr Virginia Alun Jones (Vermilion)

WOMEN'S HEALTH

A Woman's Guide to Dealing with Polycystic Ovary Syndrome, Collette
    Harris with Dr Adam Carey (Thorsons)
Natural Treatment of Fibroid Tumours and Endometriosis, Susan M.
    Lark, M.DE. (Keats Publishing)
Endometriosis – A key to healing through nutrition, Dian Shepperson
    Mills & Michael Vernon (Element Publishing)
No More PMS!, M Stewart (Vermilion)
The Breast Cancer Prevention and Recovery Diet, Suzannah Olivier
    (Michael Joseph)

Women, Hormones and the Menstrual Cycle, Ruth Trickey (Allen & Unwin)

ALLERGIES

Asthma the Complete Guide, Johnathon Brostoff & Linda Gamlin (Bloomsbury)
The Complete Guide to Food Allergy and Intolerance, Prof. Johnathon Brostoff & Linda Gamlin (Bloomsbury)

DIGESTIVE HEALTH

Superbug, Geoffrey Cannon (Virgin Publishing Ltd)
Digestive Wellness, Elizabeth Lipski (Keats Publishing)
No More IBS!, M Stewart & Dr A Stewart (Vermilion)
Overcoming Candida, Xandria Williams (Element Books)
Candida Albicans, Leon Chaitow (Inner Traditions International)

RECIPE BOOKS

SuperJuice, M. Van Straten (Mitchell Beazley)
Cook Organic, Gilli Davies (Metro Books)
Cooking Without, Barbara Cousins (Thorsons)
The Sensitive Gourmet, Antoinette Savill (Thorsons)
The Everyday Wheat Free and Gluten Free Cookbook, Michelle Berriedale-Johnson (Grub Street)
Dairy Free Cookbook, Jane Zukin (Prima)

COMPLEMENTARY THERAPIES

Qi Gong for Beginners, Stanley Wilson (Rudra Press)
The Power of Your Other Hand, Lucia Capacchione (Newcastle Publishing)
Visioning – Ten Steps to Designing the Life of Your Dreams, Lucia Capacchione (Putnam Publishing)
The Creative Journal – The Art of Finding Yourself, Lucia Capacchione (Newcastle Publishing)
Recovery of your Inner Child, Lucia Capacchione (Fireside Publishing)
Mind Power into the 21st Century, John Kehoe (Zoetic Inc. Publishing)

EXERCISE & RELAXATION

The Art of Swimming, Steven Shaw & A D'Angour (Ashgrove Publishing)

The Alexander Technique, Wilfred Barlow (Inner Traditions)
Body Control the Pilates Way, Lynne Robinson & G Thomas (Pan)
Pure Pilates, Michael King (Mitchell Beazley)

STRESS

Dynamic Yoga, Godfrey Devereux (Thorsons)
The Book of Massage, Lucy Lidell (Press)
The Book of Yoga, Sivanda Yoga Centre (Ebury Press)
Lyn Marshall's Instant Stress Cure, Lyn Marshall (Vermilion)

Index